Nursing Models for Practice

NURSING MODELS FOR PRACTICE

Alan Pearson

FRCN SRN ONC RNT DipNED MSc PhD

Senior Nurse — Clinical Practice Development
Burford Community Hospital and Nursing Development Unit
Oxfordshire Health Authority

Barbara Vaughan

SRN RCNT RNT DipN(Lond) MSc

Senior Tutor — Clinical Practice Development
John Radcliffe Hospital
Oxfordshire Health Authority

Cartoons by Kipper Williams

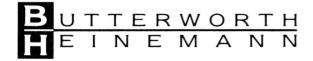

Butterworth-Heinemann Ltd
Linacre House, Jordan Hill, Oxford OX2 8DP

A member of the Reed Elsevier plc group

OXFORD   LONDON   BOSTON
MUNICH   NEW DELHI   SINGAPORE   SYDNEY
TOKYO   TORONTO   WELLINGTON

First published 1986
Reprinted 1986, 1988, 1989 (twice), 1991, 1992 (twice), 1993, 1994

ISBN 0 7506 0379 8

Printed and Bound in Great Britain at The Bath Press, Avon

Contents

Preface

This book has been written because of a recognised need among many nurses for an introductory text about nursing models. Its intention is to give an insight into what nursing models are, what their implications for practice are, and how they may be used.

A brief summary of six different models has been included to show a variety of available approaches and the way in which they can be used for patient assessment and care planning. Our aim is only to offer an introduction to this relatively new development and to give sufficient information to act as a starting point for further exploration of the subject.

Our hope is that this introduction to the application of theory to practice will in some way contribute to nursing's continuing endeavour to meet the needs of those clients and patients who require the services of nurses.

Alan Pearson and Barbara Vaughan
Oxford

Acknowledgements

This book is the product of five years' thought, reading and conversation with other nurses as well as experience in practice. So many people have contributed to its development that it would be impossible to name them all individually. All of those who deserve thanks will recognise themselves and their contribution to our thinking in the pages of the book.

We are grateful to the following for their permission to reproduce figures in the text:

The Open University
Little, Brown and Co.
Heinemann Medical Books
John Wiley & Sons Ltd.
Churchill Livingstone

Authors' note

Both of us are extremely uncomfortable about the issue of male and female pronouns in literature. We have spent considerable time discussing possible ways of overcoming this difficulty and have been unable to find a satisfactory way of referring to people in a non-sexist manner. Continually using him/her or he/she is, we feel, clumsy and does not further the cause of equality. Regretfully we have reverted to the traditional pattern of generally referring to the nurse as 'she' and the patient as 'he'. We look forward to the day when a creative writer offers a usable alternative in the English language.

1 | Models for Practice

Welcome to what we hope is a different sort of book about nursing — a book that is concerned with very basic things. At first sight these things may seem simple, but the more one thinks about them the more fascinating and complicated they become. Developing a model on which to base the practice of nursing is a very popular subject in nursing today. It is discussed widely in the nursing press, on courses for nurses and in places where nurses work. But what does this actually mean? Do we really need to spend time and energy on thinking about such things when there are so many people to be nursed, so little time and so many obstacles to be overcome in actually getting the work done? And since there is a wealth of other things to learn before we can nurse effectively, is it not better to learn skills and gain knowledge first, leaving this theorising about what nursing is and what nurses do until there is time to do so?

We believe that thinking about nursing and trying to work out a picture to represent these thoughts is the crucial beginning, not only of learning how to nurse, but also of actually nursing. This book is simply a collection of thoughts about the subject, and it takes a practical approach in order to share them with others. In the first chapter the need for using models for practice and the effects this may have on nursing care are discussed. We give a basic explanation of what a model actually is. Then these ideas are linked to the process of nursing to show how models are inextricably part of the real nursing of people.

A model — what is it?

Although the term 'model' is comparatively new in nursing, the idea is certainly not. The word 'model' is often used in everyday language. It is, of course, something which is not the real thing, but which matches or represents it as closely as possible. Those plastic models of aeroplanes given to little children (and sometimes really big children!) are certainly not capable of flying to far-away places, but the people who construct the kits try hard to make them as similar to the real thing as possible. The elaborate models constructed by architects in an attempt to explain a new building are totally unreal in terms of size, but their purpose is to faithfully represent the reality of the building. Such models are three-dimensional representations of reality made out of raw materials such as mini-bricks, metal and plastic. In contrast, models for practice, work or activity have as their raw materials ideas, beliefs, knowledge and other less tangible building bricks. But their essence is the same. The essence of models for practice will be explained later in this chapter, but it is useful to start off with a basic under-standing of a practice model — *a descriptive picture of practice which adequately represents the real thing.*

Constructing such pictures — pictures composed of ideas and values and written down in a clear way — is at first sight quite a new exercise for nurses. But of course individuals have painted such pictures about what they think is reality since the human race began. Furthermore, all nurses have a picture in their heads about what nursing actually is and what nurses do, and they base this picture on their ideas and values. Yet making such views explicit, talking and writing about them and sharing them with others, is not an activity which is commonly found among nurses.

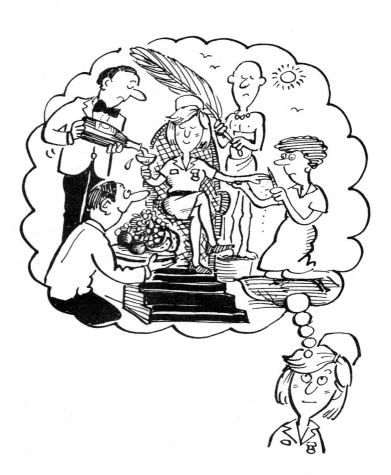

Fig. 1.1 *All nurses have pictures in their heads of what nursing actually is.*

Thus while actual models have always existed in our minds, being asked to make them explicit, to share them with others or to consider other people's views, is a new experience for most of us.

The need for models for practice

All thinking people possess views of the world, their work, and the subject of their work — in the case of nursing, the patients or clients. In occupations which involve service to other people, it gives direction to the people who work in those occupations, if they construct models from beliefs about the client and from current knowledge related to those beliefs. In teaching, for example, various writers describe teaching models which give different views about people and how they learn (e.g. Glaser, 1962; De Cecco and Crawford, 1974). Some emphasise the belief that learners need to be told clearly what the teacher requires them to know and do, and that if this happens learning will take place. Others emphasise the belief that learners themselves need to decide what they wish to know and to be able to do; they consider that learning takes place if the teacher allows this to happen and provides the resources which learners appear to need to achieve their own objectives. There are, of course, many other components to teaching models, and many other beliefs about teaching. But these two basic but different sets of beliefs, derived from two different theories of learning, serve to give an example of the need for some agreement on a model in an institution which sets out to help people learn. If the model based on setting learners objectives, and then giving them the material that is needed to achieve the objectives, is agreed on, it will give direction to the way in which the institution is run. It will influence the use of the school building, the library resources, the teaching aids and the actual behaviour of the teacher. It would probably require efficient copying facilities to print out objectives for learners, and a good stack of set texts recommended by the teachers. Alternatively, if the second model based on more active student involvement is followed, less of these facilities may be required but more private study areas and a wider selection of books would be essential.

In nursing, the care given to patients or clients is also influenced by the model held by the people who give the care. However, in very many settings, no generally agreed upon model is held. In a team of nurses, for example, one nurse may align nursing very closely with the work of doctors and aim for the efficient carrying out of medically prescribed care. In this instance less emphasis will be placed on non-medical acts such as organising social activities or transport for visitors who are unable to make their own way to hospital or to the patient's home. Another nurse may emphasise just those things and see the more medically related tasks as being important but no more so than social activities. Yet another nurse may value tidiness and order and concentrate on clean and tidy patients and ward areas. There may be one nurse who spends much time on watching and

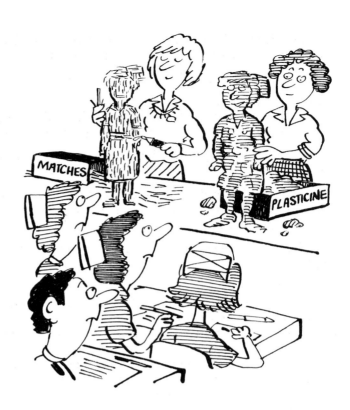

Fig. 1.2 *Personal models influence practice.*

supporting an elderly patient while she dresses herself, while another will consistently dress the patient because she sees 'doing things' for people as being a part of nursing. If you reflect on this for a moment, we suspect that it actually describes at least one area where you have worked as a nurse or seen nursing, even if you are fairly new to the work of nursing. Although all of the nurses described are fictitious and have no names, you can probably fit them to people you know. Of course all nurses are individuals and the past that belongs to them, the way they were brought up by their parents, the place they came from, and their social background as a whole, certainly influence how they behave and what they value. All of these things go towards the model for nursing practice on which they base their real work of caring for people. But some of the differences between the nurses in this fictitious team could at least be recognised. The strengths of each nurse could be better channelled if the team could somehow consider different descriptions of what nursing is and after discussion agree on generally basing practice on one, or an agreed combination of two or more, descriptions. Models of nursing practice are such descriptions. It is irrelevant which model or combination of models is agreed upon as long as agreement is reached.

Achieving agreement demands that the team as a whole consider each individual nurse's beliefs about patients and nursing work. It leads to a number of possible advantages. If a team of nurses agrees to base their practice on a generally accepted model, it will:

1. Lead to consistency in the sort of care received by patients and thus to a continuity of care patterns and treatments.

2. Give rise to less conflict within the team of nurses as a whole.

3. Make sense of the nursing given by the team; the other health care workers involved, such as doctors, physiotherapists and ancillary staff, will understand better the logic behind the care.

4. Give direction to nursing care within the area, since the goals of nursing work will be understood by the whole team.

5. Act as a major guide in decision and policy making because the components of the model chosen can act as a guide against which to check decisions.

6. Act as a guide for the criteria on which new team members are selected.

As an example, let us consider a team of nurses who all agree that the model constructed by Orem (1980) should provide a basis for practice in their work. Orem's model is described in Chapter 6. It focuses on the nurse striving to help the patient or client to care for him or herself. Thus the nurse concentrates on helping patients to do things for themselves rather than doing everything for them. If patients are unable to be independent in this way, however, nurses will act for them or on their behalf. Orem's model is, of course, more complex than this, but this specific component of it serves for this example. If self-care is the aim of nursing, patients are seen as having the right to care for themselves whenever possible. Nurses who agree to apply this model will value knowledge and skills related to promoting or giving self-care. The relationship of such a view of nursing to the six possible advantages listed above, can be demonstrated. To begin with, it can be assumed that all nurses in the team would consistently try to step back and encourage patients to do things themselves whenever possible. They would only 'do' care when the patients are unable to help themselves. Stretched to its logical conclusion, some patients may even be able to take their own medications, give their own tube feeds or dress and undress themselves, even if it takes longer than when the nurse does it. Acceptance of this by the whole team may then lessen the current situation in which patients know they will have to dress themselves when Nurse White is on duty, but will be dressed by the nurse when Nurse Green is on duty . If the self-care model is agreed upon, care will be similar all the time, with only minor variations which will always arise because of differences between individual nurses.

Less conflict may also occur because the nurse who steps back and allows patients to be independent will be less likely to be seen as lazy or slow. The other members of the health team will also begin to understand that nurses in this area all value independence as a patient's right. Because self-care is accepted as the overall goal of nursing, this will give direction to the way work is organised, to the assessment, planning, implementation and evaluation of care, and to the relationship between the nursing team and other workers. The self-care goal could be usefully used as a yardstick when decisions need to be made about issues such as choices of new equipment or alterations in drug-giving procedures. For example, when making policy decisions on how drugs should be given, options can be discussed alongside the beliefs about self-care. If two nurses are to always check drugs together and to check the patient's name-band on his wrist, does this enhance the promotion of self-care? If it does not, how can the procedure be satisfactorily modified to promote self-care?

In the event of having to choose new equipment, the choice may be between a new disposable bed-pan system or two commodes. The team may again weigh up the merits of the choice on the basis of which would be more likely to assist patients to achieve self-care.

The final point mentioned was that a model for nursing practice can be used as a guide for selecting the criteria on which a new member of staff will be appointed. If a group of nurses working together are in a position to be quite clear about the values on which they base their practice, and the goals that they are trying to achieve, there is an opportunity for both the applicant and the interviewers to discover whether they share these values and goals. Hopefully this would lessen the likelihood of someone who would not fit in being appointed to a team who have well-established views of the service that they are offering.

It is possible to go on listing all kinds of different examples, but the reasons why a team needs to agree on a model are probably becoming evident. Selecting a nursing model demands that the team agree on the nature and purpose of the work they are carrying out and on a view about the people to whom they offer that service, namely the patients or clients. *These are essential prerequisites for effective nursing.*

We could, of course, leave the system of giving care unchanged, and nurses could carry on giving care to those who need it, in the way it occurs to them to give it. However, if there are six nurses looking after one patient in a hospital ward, the chances are that the care will be based on up to six different models. Furthermore, none of these models may be appropriate for that patient. There is every likelihood that confusion will arise, leading to care which is disjointed and to a patient having to adjust to six nurses rather than to six nurses adjusting to one patient.

Actual agreement among those six nurses on a broad picture of what they consider to be the role of the nurse, the needs of the patient and what it is they are trying to achieve, will in the end lead to successful care, a satisfied patient, and a united team of nurses.

All of this may seem to be highly theoretical, and it cannot be denied that nursing is really very practical. But theory guides all practice, all living. There is an old saying that there is nothing so practical as a good theory. The practical observable movement of the car from one point to another only happened because someone

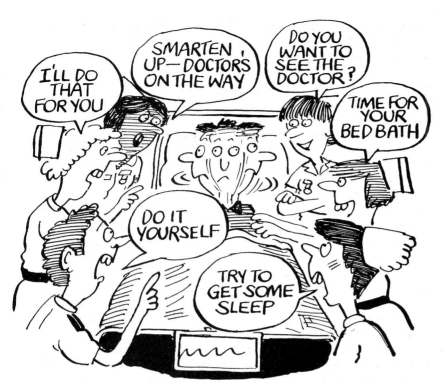

Fig. 1.3 *An agreed model stops confusion.*

worked on the theory which led to the development of the internal combustion engine.

In this book we hope to share our understanding of models in relationship to practical nursing. It is our belief that all nursing is already based on models for practice, but that at the moment nurses find it difficult to explain and share their ideas with others because they are hidden in their minds rather than explicit. The issues that need to be raised are therefore very broad, and seem at first sight to be somewhat outside what is normally considered to be important to nurses. That is why this chapter began by saying that this book is a little different. It is intended to be used both personally and professionally. On the personal level the book aims to help individual nurses to clarify their thoughts about nursing work and how they relate to it. Within ward teams or a class of students, its purpose is to promote creative thinking about developing real nursing with the help of models for practice.

Bear with us then, if these first four chapters bring up words or ideas which have been, up until now, unfamiliar or which seem inappropriate, and if the rest of the book generates more questions than clear answers. That state is the beginning of the thinking and questioning attitude which nursing demands.

The basis of models

We have already talked about the building bricks that go towards making up a nursing model. A model house constructed by an architect is made of the components of that house and represents the shapes of the rooms, the slope of the roof and the relationship of one part to another. It is not a real house, but it accurately represents reality, and the successful construction of a house is only assured if time is spent initially on the careful creation of a model. A nursing model is made up of the components or ideas which go towards making up nursing — what it is, the beliefs, the values, and the theories and the concepts on which it is built. While these words are often viewed with some caution by many people, they are in fact the building bricks of what each one of us believes nursing is. All of us already hold beliefs, have values, and understand the theories and concepts on which we base our practice. In order to be able to share our ideas with others, a brief explanation of each of these terms is necessary.

Philosophies and beliefs

Throughout the ages there have been people who have publicly stated their views about the world, about people, and about what is right and wrong. While a few have made these statements publicly, all of us do, in fact, hold such beliefs. It is these beliefs which guide the whole of our lives. Bertrand Russell wrote in 1961 that 'Ever since men became capable of free speculation, their actions in innumerable important respects have depended upon their theories as to the world and human life, as to what is good and what is evil.' From what Russell says it becomes fairly evident that what you believe about people, society and life will affect the way you behave. So philosophy can be interpreted as the pursuit of wisdom or knowledge about the things around us and what causes them. A philosophy is an explicit statement about what you believe and about what values you hold. These values and beliefs will, in turn, affect the way you behave.

Stevenson (1974) takes two well known philosophical stances, that of Christianity and of Marxism, and makes a simple comparison of them to demonstrate this point. The Christian view of people is that they are made in the image of God, who created and controls the universe. The goal or purpose of human lives is to fulfil God's purpose and their state is dependent on their relationship with God. On the other hand, Marx suggested that the universe is fundamentally material and that nothing exists beyond it.

Our moral ideas and values are determined by the society in which we live. If the Christian belief is followed, the way forward lies in God's ability to forgive and regenerate in His image. The Marxist view, however, holds that an individual cannot change without fundamental changes in society. Two people holding these opposing views will ultimately behave in quite different ways — one seeking to develop in the image of God and the other seeking to change society in order to influence the way individuals behave.

Take a concrete example with which we are all familiar. We have already said that there are two different views about how we learn, and our experience of 'being taught' clearly confirms this. There is the teacher who will stand before a class and lecture, who will 'deposit' a body of information for us to absorb because he or she believes that as the holder of expert knowledge on a given subject, his or her role is to hand on this knowledge to others. This is something we have all experienced at some time in our educational careers. Alternatively, there are those teachers who believe that people learn more effectively if they discover things for themselves. Their approach may be through guiding seminars prepared by learners, and through involvement and discussion with very active participation on the part of the whole group. One explanation for these two different styles of teaching is that the beliefs of the two types of teachers are based on completely different theories of learning, namely expository learning and discovery learning, which are derived from different philosophies or beliefs.

In the same way, we are all familiar with nurses who behave in different ways in the same situation. A currently topical example is the nurse's feelings about the use of high technology medicine for very elderly patients with the aim to preserve life at all costs. One group of nurses will consider that, whatever the circumstances, if such treatment is available it should be given. Another view may be that the use of such treatment depends upon the individual circumstances of each patient, and that patients have a right to choose whether or not to receive treatment which in itself may be traumatic, their decision being based on their own views about the quality of their lives. The argument may be seen as being related to quantity versus quality. It is fundamentally based on a belief system about nature and life itself.

In talking about philosophies, it becomes evident that they are made up of the views or ideas about the subject being discussed. Relating this to nursing, there are two questions that have to be asked. First, what are the specific subjects which we need to consider and clarify in relationship to nursing? And, second, what ideas or theories do we hold in relationship to these subjects?

Concepts

A concept of a particular subject is the way in which it is viewed. It is a classification system applied to a particular area. Yet not all of us would classify things in the same way. This becomes very obvious when you try to find your way through a colleague's filing system and end up saying in exasperation 'I'd never have put it there'. Yet to the person who established the filing system, it is the obvious place. *As cells are units of the body, so concepts are units of the mind.*

Nursing itself may be seen as a very large collection of concepts, as made up of numerous concepts: those things which individuals consider are important to nursing, those things which nurses need to know about and to develop theories about. It may be worthwhile to stop here for a minute and consider what major concepts you think are related to nursing. Hopefully they will be very similar to the ones identified by the people with whom you work. Otherwise there may be terrible confusion in trying to find your way about the filing system of each other's thoughts.

The most commonly identified concepts which have been discussed in relationship to nursing are those relating to beliefs about people, society, health and nursing itself. A philosophy of nursing usually makes statements about each of these subjects.

Theories

The next stage of the game is to try and work out how the concepts fit together in practice, and this is the stage at which theories have to be considered. Theories are proposals which give a reasonable explanation to an event. They are ideas about how or why something happens. Returning to the example of teaching that we gave earlier, there are two different theories about how people learn — neither of which is proved absolutely. Once proved beyond reasonable doubt, a theory is considered to be a law. Until that time individuals must make knowledgeable judgements about the theories they accept, and they need where possible to test their theories or to support them by facts. With the passage of time and the advancement of knowledge, theories may change and develop.

An example of this is that previously there was a theory in nursing that rubbing skin vigorously prevented the formation of pressure sores. With the advancement of time, and with it the acquisition of new knowledge, it became known that this theory is inaccurate and that in fact rubbing is potentially harmful. So new theories, based on an understanding of the anatomy and physiology of skin and the circulation of blood, have been proposed and widely accepted. Similarly, with new knowledge about the nature of people and views of health, theories about what nursing is and how it may be practised have developed.

There are two ways in which theories can be developed. First, someone may come up with an idea and wonder whether it is related to practice. For instance, with the current interest in complementary or, as they are more commonly known, alternative therapies, the question of whether or not they are of any value to nurses, and through them to patients, may be asked. This type of theory is known as a deductive theory. It takes ideas which are already established in other fields and considers ways in which they may be related to nursing practice. Theories from both the physical and behavioural sciences have been applied to nursing in this way. For example, theories about bonding between parents and children have been applied in a deductive way and have altered the practice of nursing in both obstetrics and paediatrics.

Alternatively, it may be observed through practice that patients in one situation seem to recover more quickly than patients in another, and a nurse may set out to find out if this is true. This is known as an inductive theory, that is a theory that arises out of practice. Inductive theory building does not depend on an already established theory, but involves generating new ideas through exploring practice, identifying concepts and relating them to establish a new theory. For example, close observation of people approaching death led to the identification of recognised stages through which people progress at this time. On first learning of impending death, people react with feelings of shock, denial and isolation. This may be followed by feelings of anger. The third phase is one of bargaining, during which people tend to ask 'why me?'. A depressive phase is often experienced after this. Recognition of these phases assists nurses in helping people to progress through them to a final stage of acceptance which may lead to either resignation or to a fight to the last (Kübler-Ross, 1969). Both approaches are equally valid and necessary for the advancement of practice.

Returning to models for nursing and the way in which nurses practise, the very foundations of these models and approaches to practice lie in an individual's philosophy or beliefs about nursing. This in turn is based on how each individual classifies nursing and the subjects related to it, as well as the theories believed to be true. Over a period of time every nurse has developed such a model. The time has come to be explicit about these thoughts and to be able to share them with others.

Components of models

The notion that what nurses believe in actually affects the way in which they behave has been emphasised throughout this chapter. The model of nursing on which practice is based contains the theories and concepts of that practice, and the theories and concepts reflect the philosophies, values and beliefs about both human nature and what it is that nursing is trying to achieve. With these points in mind, there are three basic components of any practice model:

1. The beliefs and values on which the model is based.

2. The goals of practice or what the practitioner aims to achieve.

3. The knowledge and skills the practitioner needs to develop in order to gain these goals.

There are similarities in any model of an occupation like teaching or nursing where the subject of practice is a person rather than an object.

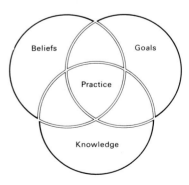

Fig. 1.4 *Components of a model for practice.*

Beliefs and values

Any occupation concerned with the provision of a human service has to adopt a stance about the nature of people and how they behave. This stance will underpin any model of that occupation. And, because people do not exist in isolation but as part of a community and of society itself, the issues of community and society must also be considered. Just as a carpenter must understand the nature of wood, his essential raw material — of how pliable or durable it is and how it reacts with other materials — so any person who is dealing with a human service must have some understanding of how people, or the recipients of their service, function.

Compared to the complexity of human nature, wood is a relatively simple subject, and there are many confirmed facts or laws about the way in which it will behave. For example, it is indisputable that unseasoned wood will alter its shape in a fairly predictable way as it matures. Remember the squeaking floorboards when unseasoned wood has been used!

The huge range of individual differences among people makes it impossible for those whose work is with them to be anywhere near as certain about all aspects of human behaviour as a carpenter can be about his wood. There are no such things as 'truths' about human nature. However, there are many theories which give different explanations of it and in any occupation or discipline which involves practice, particular theories are adopted as beliefs on which to base the practice. Different occupations focus on specific aspects of humanity according to the service they offer. For example, teaching models will always focus on beliefs about how people learn. In sociology the emphasis is on how people relate to each other and in psychology on how they behave. Health care has traditionally emphasised the biological aspect of human beings. Current thoughts are challenging this tradition.

The beliefs and values component of the practice model are the foundations on which the whole of the rest of the model is built. They influence all practice.

Goals of practice

Returning to the example of carpenters, their goals or what they expect to achieve are usually quite clear. For instance, at the start of their work, they will already have an idea about the size, design and finish of the chairs that they are trying to produce.

It is equally important in providing a service to patients that the overall purpose of the service is made clear to the practitioner and to the consumer of the service — in the case of nursing, the client or patient. This second component of the model therefore demands that the occupational group agree on the common purpose towards which it is striving.

Again because there is so much variety among individuals, there may be some variation in the recognised goals. For instance, some teachers may see their goal as ensuring that the learner has sufficient knowledge to pass an examination. Others may identify a broader goal of helping learners to solve their own problems and to develop skills for a particular work situation. This of course is often overcome by educational institutes opting to aim for 'learning to take place' and leaving it to individual practitioners to decide on how to achieve that goal.

The goals of human service occupations are strongly influenced by social expectations and they rarely remain static. The traditional goals of health care have been to cure and there is evidence that this is still true. However, practitioners and consumers alike are now increasingly calling for a wider view of the goals of health care.

Knowledge and skills for practice

Just as the goals of practice arise from the beliefs and values adopted by the occupation, the knowledge and skills needed by practitioners are determined by the stated goals of the model. Once a discipline which involves practice has identified its beliefs and values and what it is trying to achieve, it becomes relatively easy to identify the knowledge and skills required for the practice.

Returning to the carpenter, if there is a belief that wood is a material which can be changed, and that through carving and fitting it can be made into a chair, then the carpenter must have knowledge about the properties of wood, and he must have skill in using the tools required to make a chair. To find out what knowledge and which skills are required for a practice discipline (an occupation which gives a service to people), it is useful to consider the discipline's beliefs about humans and the goals of the discipline. In traditional health care, the basic views have been related to the belief in people as biological creatures who can be affected by disease, and the goals have been grounded in a desire to cure. This has therefore led to a need for knowledge based on the biological sciences and disease, supported by technical skills to administer treatment.

If it is recognised that there are alternatives to these beliefs and goals, then inevitably there must be alternative or additional knowledge and skills required for practice.

Any model for practice must contain these three basic components — beliefs and values, goals of practice, and the knowledge and skills needed to reach those goals — and all of us actually possess a personal model of this kind. A nursing model is the application of this structure to nursing itself. It enables nurses to make explicit the way in which they work.

The nursing process and nursing models

A nursing model is a picture or representation of what nursing actually is. In fact it represents the actual 'goods' which are delivered to the client. All goods, however, need some vehicle through which they are delivered and the nursing process serves this function. The process itself says nothing about the content and is not specific to nursing. It is merely a sequence of steps passed through in order to achieve a desired end, and it can be seen in use by many other occupational groups.

As can be seen in Figure 1.5, nursing is a package of goods which is to be delivered. The process of assessment, planning, implementation and evaluation are merely the delivery vehicles responsible for ensuring that the package arrives safely. The package, or nursing itself, is the model which guides the process and contains the components of which nursing is made. Each without the other is of little use to the patients.

This first chapter has explored the notion of models for practice and expanded some of the underlying issues. The influences that beliefs and values have on practice and the relationship of theories and concepts to practice have been discussed. The manner in which these underlying issues affect the components of the model have also been highlighted alongside what are considered to be the basic components of any model of an occupation which gives a service to people. While it is recognised that some of these issues are not normally discussed by nurses, it is hoped that their relevance has become clear. Being explicit about the model on which nursing practice is based in a particular setting directly affects the delivery of nursing care to patients. Its importance cannot be denied.

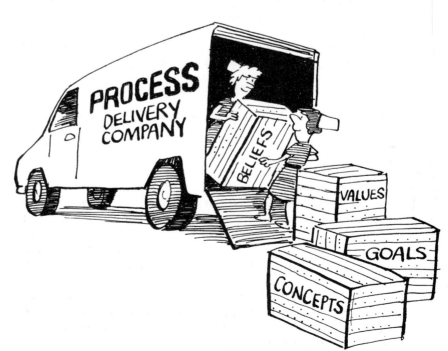

Fig. 1.5 *The nursing process is a vehicle for the delivery of care.*

2 | The Traditional Model for Nursing Practice

All nurses — all people — hold a model for practice, and although the term model may be new, basing practice on a model has occurred since nursing began.

It is argued by many that the basic model which guides nursing has traditionally been the medical model. This 'biomedical' model has also traditionally been the basis for the practice of medicine in the Western world for the last few hundred years. Before describing this long-standing model, it is important to emphasise that it has been the subject of some criticism over the years, that it is rejected in part by many doctors today and that a number of doctors practise from a much broader base. However, the medical establishment and the majority of medical schools still see the biomedical model as an accurate representation of the reality of doctoring.

Following the outline of the model presented in Chapter 1, the biomedical model can be summarised into three basic components — namely beliefs and values, the goals of practice, and the knowledge needed to achieve these goals.

The beliefs and values which underlie the biomedical model

In this model human beings are seen as biological beings, made up of cells, which then make tissues, which then make organs, which then make systems. All of these interact and communicate with each other to achieve harmony or balance, a state called homeostasis. Biological homeostasis is seen as health and is a state which is achievable but which can be disturbed by trauma, malfunction or malformation. Such disturbance leads to disease or 'medical conditions'. Although this is the core belief of the model, and human beings are in part regarded almost like machines, development of the model in recent years has led to some acknowledgement of social and psychological disturbances of homeostasis. However, the emphasis remains on biological homeostasis and the physical signs and manifestations of it. The physical working parts of the person are of prime importance.

The goals of the biomedical model

Medical practice ultimately aims for biological homeostasis, the curing or control of disease, or the repair of trauma or malformation. The goal can be achieved by diagnosing the cause of disturbed homeostasis and treating it. When cure is impossible, the goal can be modified to either alleviating the manifestations of the disturbance, in other words treating the symptoms, or to postponing death.

The knowledge needed to achieve the goals of the biomedical model

In order to diagnose and to treat disease or trauma by administering specific treatments, the practitioner needs knowledge about the physical sciences and skills to recognise physical signs and symptoms. Such knowledge would therefore arise from concepts and theories related to the physical sciences, for example:

- Anatomy
- Physiology
- Biochemistry
- Pharmacology
- Pathology
- Microbiology

The knowledge and skills focus on the physical being, and the gamut of 'faults' which may arise in the continuous functioning of the body must be included.

Nursing and the biomedical model

There is a great deal of evidence to suggest that the biomedical model is the model on which many nurses base their practice. Research studies in nursing frequently report on how nurses continue to view patients as physical beings and pay little attention to the wider characteristics of human nature. They also suggest that the goals of nursing are frequently perceived as being cure orientated and that feelings of failure often arise in nurses when cure is not achieved. The commentaries on nursing by sociologists and other non-nurses, which are based on observation, all support these suggestions and discuss the very common atmosphere of routines, standardised activity and nurses' obsession with giving physical care.

Routinisation

British nursing is often based on the prescribed routine which is frequently laid down in the policy or procedure books which are strategically placed in each ward. These rules have traditionally been created by a hierarchy of nurses who see it as their responsibility to ensure that the rules are adhered to. The end result of such an approach is standardised routines for patient care. The patient is seen as someone who should comply to a predictable pattern and follow the routine laid down by the regulations. Such routines are usually related to the medical diagnosis of the patient.

For example, there is an expectation that all people undergoing abdominal hysterectomy will walk to the bathroom on the first day postoperatively and will not require intramuscular analgesia after the second day. Such routines focus primarily on the diagnostic label. They depersonalise patients and discourage any close involvement between them and nurses, because the patients are identified as the possessors of a disease process rather than as individuals. They become known as 'the appendix in bed 6' and not Mrs Smith, a wife and a mother and a woman with a life of her own.

The classic biomedical model focuses on correctly diagnosing disease — the nurse's role being to accurately carry out medical prescriptions. Establishing routines to ensure that this happens is a natural result of adherence to the medical model. For instance, administration of analgesia at the same time each day, regardless of individual preferences, would be seen as good practice in these circumstances.

While some routines can be valuable and necessary — such as the safety measures to be followed preoperatively — their wider use not only depersonalises care but is also potentially dangerous and wasteful of time. The unnecessary recording of observations or the two-hourly turning of all bedridden patients are examples of a waste of the precious resource of nursing time. Furthermore, the imposition of routine practices such as a daily recording of Norton scores for all patients has not been found to be helpful. In a recent study it was found that the prescription and practice of nursing in relationship to the care of the pressure areas did not relate in any way to the Norton score which had been routinely recorded.

Physical care

Routinisation is often accompanied by an obsession with physical care. Because the biomedical model focuses on people as physical beings, nurses who base their practice on it concentrate on the person's physical needs. Value is placed on those visible aspects of care such as cleanliness, prompt fulfilment of treatment and pre-scriptions, and tidy beds, cupboards and ward areas. Technical skills such as recording of electrocardiograms or taking intravenous blood are given more status than the ability to comfort distressed people or to share information with those who have little under-standing of their own situation. The priority of care based on the biomedical model is always towards excellence in physical care, and other components of care are either left unrecognised or not seen as being important. However, both an obsession with physical care and routinisation have been said to be useful strategies in protecting nurses against the stress inherent in their work. Together they mean that nurses can maintain a distance from patients and not concern themselves with anything other than the disease process, physical care and the maintenance of a routine.

Getting the work done

'Getting through the work' is usually the major goal of nursing teams in the health service, and this is directly related to the emphasis of the biomedical model. There is little attention paid to the meeting of needs of people as individuals. High value is placed on nurses who are able to complete certain defined tasks before handing over to the next nurse on duty. The emphasis is again placed on completion of the visible tasks which are associated with physical care and routines. Since this is the mechanism used for setting priorities within the work environment, little or no time is left at the end of the day for the personalised aspects of care.

Care versus cure

The overriding goal of the biomedical model is cure and therefore nurses who base their practice on it also aim for this outcome. This causes confusion and problems for nurses who work in fields where a 'cure' is not possible. For example, uncertainty as to whether curing or caring is the goal of practice has been observed in long-stay psychiatric wards, young disabled units, mental handicap units and in the institutional and community care of the elderly — all areas where the patients cannot 'recover' or get 'completely better'. Nurses working in these units are consistently faced with an inability to achieve the outcome of care that they believe to be appropriate, that is to cure. Death, or failure to cure, represents a failure in itself and the nurses as a consequence may become dissatisfied in their work.

If the orientation of the care-giver is towards cure, the manner in which care is provided will reflect this, laying stress on activities which relate to cure, rather than on providing an environment in which individualised care can be delivered.

The emphasis of cure as a general goal of nursing is still reflected today in the difficulties that are experienced in staffing units which care for chronically dependent people. It is also seen in continuing education, where competition is intense for places on courses associated with complex technical care directed at cure, such as the intensive care or accident and emergency courses, whereas places on courses concerned with care of the elderly are more easily attained.

If it is believed that nursing should be available to anyone who is in need of nursing care, then the biomedical model is no longer an appropriate basis for practice. It is limiting because it confines nursing to those who can achieve cure, and it creates a dilemma for nurses who work with those people for whom a cure is unattainable.

The knowledge and skills given to nurses in their professional training, at least until very recently, have been structured around the beliefs inherent in the medical model. The curriculum revolved around anatomy, physiology, pathology and other physical sciences, although at a much lower academic level than medical training. It included very little, if any, specified learning about the social, environmental and psychological components of human beings. This meant that just as in practice the doctors based their assessment, planning, care giving and evaluation on a framework structured around the systems of the body, so did nurses. There is strong evidence from current and on-going research that this pattern of nursing still prevails.

Professional training and experience are not the only factors that determine the models of practice held by nurses. Nurses are individuals and will therefore always incorporate additional beliefs, goals and knowledge specific to themselves. However, the essence of each person's own model is profoundly influenced by the commonly shared model held by the professional group. While it is reasonable for us to assume that most nurses do operate from the perspective of the biomedical model, most nurses also expand it to include other beliefs and some use a very different approach. Nurses who strongly identify with the biological–physical view of human beings and the goal of cure in their work may also take into account the individual differences between people. Nevertheless the focus may be on physical aspects and this will take precedence over other aspects of the person.

Evolution of the biomedical model

The most influential model for practice in health care over the last century has been this so-called 'biomedical model', and it is both interesting and relevant to look briefly at its development as an understanding of what has gone before is invaluable for planning what is to come. Pietroni (1984), in writing of his commitment to holistic medicine, gives a succinct account of the evolution of the biomedical model.

It was with the explosion of knowledge which took place in the Renaissance that the major split between religion and science occurred — prior to that time thinking had been strongly influenced by the belief that all actions were divinely controlled. René Descartes, a great philosopher of the Renaissance put forward the concept of *dualism*, of a mind free from external forces and able to think logically and independently. Thus he separated the body from the mind. He viewed the body as a machine capable of malfunction if some of the parts were not working, and suggested that the most effective way of studying this body or machine was to break it down into its component parts in order that the malfunctioning of each part could be identified and corrected.

This philosophical view was to influence the way in which science, and in particular the science of heath care, progressed over the next three hundred years. The mind and soul became the province of the clerics, while the body became the province of the doctor. As knowledge progressed, the body was split into ever smaller parts — first systems, then organs, then tissues and then

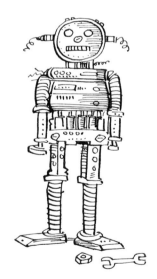

Fig. 2.1 *Some people view the body as a machine capable of malfunction.*

cells. This approach, known as the *reductionist* approach, has been invaluable in the achievement of scientific knowledge and has led to enormous knowledge about the management of disorders which affect the body. It is easily recognised in our current society by the innumerable specialities concerned only with a small part of the whole person. The contribution of specialists must never be underestimated since their knowledge and skills have led to the alleviation of immeasurable suffering in human beings. But it is out of these views that the biomedical model grew, viewing people as being made up of many parts, each of which was studied independently. The fight to cure or control disease is easily recognised as the goal. The ever more complex technical knowledge must also be recognised and valued, according to this model.

The biomedical view remained largely unchallenged until recent times, and its influence can be seen not only in medicine but also in the way in which nursing has evolved. The dictionary definition of nursing says that it is concerned not only with nourishment but also with care for the decrepit or sick. Western society has always recognised the need for such a service and nurses have always existed in one form or another. In early days the nursing role was largely carried out in the community by lay people, but nursing was also to be found in religious institutions. Bevis (1978) describes the underlying value of these religious institutions as *asceticism*, the dedicated individual committing his or her life to the care of others and providing the basic needs of food, shelter and comfort. Asceticism is associated with denial of one's own needs in order to serve others. It was demonstrated by a total commitment; the person lived within the institution where care was provided, dissociated from the outside world. Remnants of such an approach are still visible in old hospital buildings where the matrons' living quarters were within the hospital building and the sisters' rooms still provide a convenient meeting place for some staff within the confines of the ward itself.

However, a review of the popular literature concerned with life in the eighteenth and nineteenth centuries also reveals another kind of nurse, the Sarah Gamps of this world, so vividly described by Dickens, with a greater love of the gin bottle than the patient. Nursing took on the cloak of refuge for many who were near destitution themselves.

It was the influence of Florence Nightingale, and some of her contemporaries, such as Bedford Fenwick of the late nineteenth century, who were to change much of this. It can be argued that Florence Nightingale sought to make nursing 'respectable' and one way in which she achieved this was to firmly attach it to medicine, describing the function of nursing as carrying out what doctors said was required for the care of the patient.

The inevitable result of this was a strong influence on the value systems, goals and knowledge of nursing. While the ascetic value of early days persisted, new values were taken on board. Bevis again describes this, first as *romanticism*, with a hero worship of the

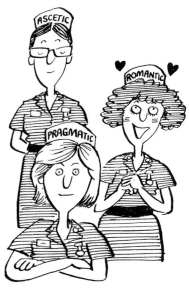

Fig. 2.2 *Asceticism, romanticism and pragmatism have been important values in nursing.*

leader or doctor and a subservient relationship to him. With the burst of technology of the 1940s and 1950s, romanticism lost favour and she suggests that the overruling value became *pragmatism*, the skilled technical nurse extending her role to cope with the direct effects of new technical knowledge.

Pragmatism is associated with a practical approach to assessing situations and acting on them. It tests things by their practical consequences. Since the underlying value system of nursing at this time was associated with disease and cure, the skills that were developed were also linked to them. The special courses that were developed, for example by the Joint Board of Clinical Nursing Studies, helped nurses to attain the specific practical skills associated with increased medical technology. Some acknowledgement was given to other aspects of care, but the emphasis lay on deepening the understanding of disease processes, their physical effects and their technical management.

While the importance of such technical skills is in no way underestimated, many people are now asking whether some of the essence of nursing has been lost through an over-emphasis on them.

The reductionist approach that so strongly influenced medicine has played its part in nursing too. An understanding of the origins of many of the complementary paramedical groups such as physiotherapists, occupational therapists and social workers clearly demonstrates that their roots lie in nursing. The splits have also occurred with nursing itself and many 'specialist' nurses have emerged with detailed and expert knowledge about particular aspects of their subject. The value of such people is immense, but as in so many situations, there is always a price to pay for such skills. The risks in this case are two-fold. First, it has led to a loss of some skills by the 'ordinary' nurse. Somewhere the task of helping a

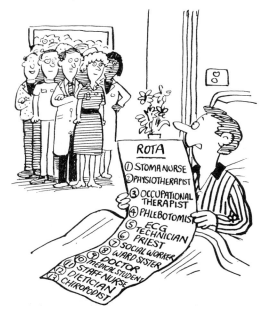

Fig. 2.3 *The consequences of the reductionist approach.*

patient to dress independently has been lost to occupational therapists, of encouraging mobility to physiotherapists, and of stoma care to stoma therapists. The patient has been split into many parts, his or her needs for each separate function being met by either specialist nurses who have extended their role in one particular direction or by relatively new occupational groups who have taken over some functions previously carried out by nurses.

The trend toward specialisation complies with the original thoughts of Descartes many hundreds of years ago. It has led to many advantages, particularly a deeper knowledge and understanding of specific areas of care and the availability of expert knowledge. Yet in some areas the biomedical model and the divisions and specialisations it leads to are now being challenged. Many people from both nursing and medicine are asking whether alternative approaches may be more appropriate and are seeking ways of meeting people's health care needs more effectively. Hence the emergence of alternative models of nursing, described by nurses for nursing. These models show nursing to have a unique and separate function in its own right.

Influences of the biomedical model on practice

There is no doubt that the biomedical model has, and still does, influence the practice of nursing, and we can observe how its ideas have actually affected nursing as a service.

A model is based on values and attitudes; in turn, a model influences what will be valued and what will be seen as being of more or less status or worth. The biomedical model values knowledge about the physical sciences and the performance of treatment activities which will lead to diagnosis or cure. This is reflected strongly in nursing today. At the ward or community level, nursing activities associated with diagnosis and treatment, which are also very often of a technical nature, are frequently seen as being of a higher status than those which relate to comfort and cleanliness. Those concerned with emotion and pleasure are of even less status. Importantly, this hierarchy of valued activities also extends to a hierarchy of roles in nursing.

The 'higher-up nurse' is expected to perform the cure-directed acts such as giving drugs, performing surgical dressings and so on. The 'lower-down nurse' will give the physical care activities, such as bathing or giving bedpans. The psychosocial care is given by anyone at all — if there is time to do it. If there is no time for the psychosocial care, it can be safely left undone because not only is it invisible but it is also perceived as being of less importance. Such a hierarchy of tasks and roles is one of the reasons why the method of work organisation we often call task assignment or allocation became so popular and why it is still very much the dominant method used by nurses.

On a broader level, types of nursing that are valued are determined by the priorities set by the biomedical model. Nurses who

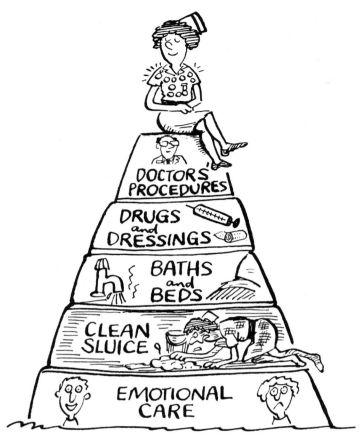

Fig. 2.4 *The hierarchy of tasks and roles in nursing.*

work in high technology units or acute hospital wards have traditionally been afforded higher status. Furthermore, until very recently, these areas tended to attract the 'best' nurses, and nurses working in these areas were assured of good career progression. Nursing in a geriatric unit, in a long-stay psychiatric hospital, in district nursing and in other non-cure areas was regarded with lower esteem, and these areas were thought of as the places where the less-bright nurse who could not cope or had blotted her copybook ended up. Although they are less common, such attitudes still exist. For example, incidents still occur where nurses who are brought before a disciplinary hearing are then transferred as a punitive measure or demotion to work in a geriatric ward.

The biomedical model, therefore, has led to an emphasis on the technical, medically-related aspects of the nursing role and to a resulting devaluation of acts related to how individuals are experiencing their own illnesses or disabilities, such as listening, comforting or the offering of choices. It also creates confusion and dissatisfaction about nursing roles such as the health visitor's role which are not involved with diagnosing and treating disease, and it leads to divisions and separatist movements within the occupation of nursing itself.

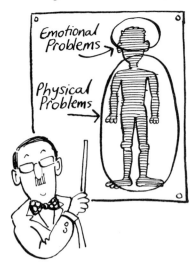

Fig. 2.5 *The biomedical model separates the mind from the body.*

The biomedical model is a well-developed one, and undoubtedly it at least gives direction to practice which is, in itself, useful. Its concentration on objectivity and efficiency was instrumental in developing nursing from the body of relatively unskilled and uneducated women mentioned earlier, to an army of highly efficient workers who are crucial to any effective health care service. If the biomedical model is accepted by a nursing team as the appropriate framework on which to base practice and all agree to pursue it, then it will, as will any other model, give direction to the care given, ensure that the care is consistent and outline the requirements for effective care.

However, the biomedical model is reductionist and dualistic in approach — it both reduces the human body to a set of related parts and it separates the mind from the body — and its common use in nursing is no longer appropriate. It is not geared to the needs of individuals and its dominant effect on health care has led to it being used in the interest of health professionals rather than those who seek, need or are directed to health care. Therefore it can no longer be acknowledged as a possible choice when nursing teams are selecting a model for their practice.

Making the choice about what model to use depends on two major considerations: the feelings of the individuals involved and the advantages and disadvantages of the model. It is therefore useful to end this discussion of the biomedical model by looking at its advantages and disadvantages.

Advantages and disadvantages of the biomedical model

Many people will argue that the biomedical model is the most efficient and effective one for use by health care workers. Some of the arguments that are put forward include:

1. The overriding concern of the patient is for cure and control of his or her disease and this model gives clear direction in this respect.

2. The knowledge base it uses is developed from scientific experiment and in many instances is objective and proved beyond reasonable doubt.

3. Since the focus of the model is disease, there is no question but that it is the doctor who should ultimately be responsible for controlling all health care. Thus any confusion or disagreement over management, whether arising from the patient/client or other health care workers, can be overruled by the doctor.

4. Its value has been proved over the years and because of this it is non-threatening and understood by both patients and health care workers alike.

5. Since it limits itself to the physical domain, the less objective psychosocial areas can be ignored.

Regardless of the fact that these arguments have withstood the test of time, alternative views are now being raised more and more frequently. It is not only health care workers but patients themselves who are raising objections to the biomedical model. Some of these are as follows:

1. There is an expectation with the biomedical model that nurses will be the humanisers of care. This expectation is often unmet.

2. The biomedical model leads to patients being labelled with a diagnosis rather than being known as a person. Patients dislike this.

3. The biomedical model's emphasis on high technology leads to the loss of human care. Both health care workers and patients are dissatisfied with this.

4. The biomedical model concentrates information and decision-making in the hands of doctors and, to a lesser extent, of other health professionals. Patients should have the right to have information about their own health and some degree of choice in its management.

Capra (1982) suggests that the biomedical model demands that the doctor hold the power in all decision-making and, as a result, '. . . the important role that nurses play in the healing process through their healing contacts with the patient is not fully recognised'. In other words, the human side of health care is devalued.

It is not our intention to either recommend or condemn this model to you. We present it as the traditional model on which practice was based for many years and commend it for the contribution it has made in the past. However, as a basis for nursing practice it can no longer be considered appropriate. Both pressure from society and increased understanding of human nature have high-lighted the restrictive nature of the biomedical model in terms of nursing practice, and alternative approaches are crucial to the provision of a satisfactory nursing service for patients.

3

Common Characteristics of Nursing Models — The Patient or Client

Many models for practice have been developed specifically for nursing. Many of these have been published and they are mainly by American writers. All of the models have different focuses, but equally they all have many ideas in common. This chapter explores the three major theories on which nursing models are based. It also examines one of the features common to models of nursing and that is the patient or client. Considering basic theories and common features in this way means that specific models can be described more easily in later chapters.

As was mentioned at the beginning of this book, theory is often a little tedious and boring at first sight, and its relevance to real, live, practical nursing is not always immediately apparent. Much of this next chapter is made up of theory and may therefore need to be read more than once. Certainly we had great difficulty when first facing this kind of material. However, over the years we have personally come to find it very meaningful to the real nursing care given. The theories and concepts we are about to provide you with are, we feel, knowledge which is fundamental to the eventual practical application of nursing models, whether in a ward or community nursing setting. Learning about them is not easy and many nurses, including us, find this prelude to learning about models difficult. We cannot apologise for this, but we do urge you to press on with these chapters, re-reading them until they are meaningful.

All models for any discipline draw on theories and concepts. Three major theories have come to be recognised as having relevance to nursing — systems theory, developmental theory and interactionist theory. Some models focus mainly on one of these theories, some combine two of them or all three, but all models include the essence of all of them in some way or another. Despite their apparent complexity, it is important to be familiar with the core of these three theories.

Systems theory

The idea of systems is one which is familiar to most nurses. The gastrointestinal system or the cardiovascular system are frequently talked about. Systems are also recognised in other walks of life — a filing system, a system of government or a computer system. People can also be described as systems.

There are particular characteristics which have been ascribed to things in order that they can be called systems. They usually have a common purpose. For example, the common purpose of the filing system may be seen as storage of documents. The parts of a system are interrelated and interdependent. Thus in the case of the cardiovascular system, the rate and pressure at which the blood is circulated is dependent on the strength of the muscular activity of the heart. Similarly the force of contraction of the heart is dependent on the flow of blood through that organ. Both responses aim to maintain homeostasis.

All systems have boundaries which can be defined, in some cases more clearly than in others. Thus the boundary of a filing system can be clearly seen as the exterior cabinet, while the boundary of a government system is less easily defined.

In all systems theory there is an emphasis on the interaction of the parts to form the whole. Each part can and should be studied separately, but functionally what is most important is the interaction of the parts and the eventual output or end result.

Two types of systems have traditionally been described. A closed system is one where the boundary does not allow for any interaction of the parts of the system with stimuli from the environment in which it exists. In reality some people suggest that there is no such thing as a closed system since everything interacts with its environment.

An open system is one which can constantly interact with its environment through its boundary. There is an input to the system, an internal rearrangement of the system and feedback. Thus in the filing system the input may be a new document. This in turn will lead to some movement of the files to make room for it. The output or end result will be a retrievable document. Some people have described the cardiovascular system as a 'closed system', but in fact it is constantly interacting with its environment, responding to hormonal changes within the body, temperature changes in the immediate environment, and emotional changes.

The characteristics of systems theory can be summarised as:

1. Systems seek to exist in a steady state, in a state of equilibrium where the parts of the system are in balance.

2. The parts of a system continually interrelate and interact with one another.

3. Each system has a boundary which is more clearly defined in some cases than in others.

4. A system can be affected by stresses occurring either within the whole system or external to the system but crossing its boundaries.

WHOLE SYSTEM

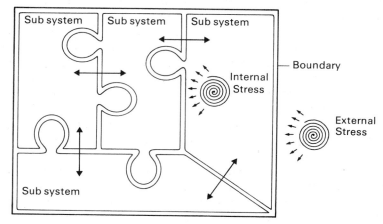

A whole system
-has parts which are interdependent
-has a clear boundary
-is affected by internal/external stresses
-seeks to maintain a balance

Fig. 3.1.

5. A stress will lead to a feedback in the system causing change in the balance. This may be temporary or require a permanent change.

6. Systems can be described as 'closed' or 'open'. In closed systems the boundary is tight and cannot be crossed. In open systems the boundary is easily crossed or affected by external stimuli.

The majority of health care models are in fact based on systems theory, and the variations that occur between models are in the perceived boundaries of the system. The biomedical model is inclined to take each body system as an entity in its own right. However, in models of nursing, the whole system that is most usually taken is of human beings in their entirety. Thus people themselves are systems made up of sub-systems and living in a supra-system.

If a change occurs in one sub-system, it will mean that the balance between all sub-systems will be disrupted and this will have an impact on the whole organisation. The response to such a disruption or stress will be to seek to return to the previous state in order to restore the balance or equilibrium. If this is not possible then a new state of equilibrium must be sought. For instance, a broken leg will not only cause changes in the musculoskeletal sub-system but will have an effect on all the other sub-systems that make up the person. However, it is likely to heal and the previous state of equilibrium will be restored. If the leg is amputated, there will be no opportunity of seeking to return to the previous state of balance, and a new one must be found.

Just as changes in the sub-systems of people will influence them as a whole, so changes in the supra-system, those systems that make up the immediate and distant environment, will also have their effect. A change in the social circumstances surrounding the individual will cause 'stresses' which will cross the boundaries of the whole system — that is the whole person. Again the changes may be temporary, causing a temporary imbalance in the whole system. For instance, an acute episode of illness will mean a temporary change in an individual's ability to earn a living. However, if the illness or disorder is of a permanent nature, as with the amputee, a permanent change in the way in which the individual reacts to the environment will have to be found.

The influence of systems theory is evident in the majority of nursing models. The whole system is usually seen as the human being. There is however, considerable variation in the way in which the systems are described. Roper *et al.* (1980) use activities of living as their framework. Roy (1976) uses the concept of stress or stimuli and the way in which humans adapt to them in four different modes — physical, self-concept, role function and interdependence. The influence of systems theory can also be seen in the traditional medical model.

Developmental theory

A second major organising theory which can be found in some nursing models is that of development. Developmental models centre around growth and change. The growth and change occur in recognised stages, are caused by identifiable variables and move in a predictable direction. While developmental theory may focus on growth, the theory can also be applied to a movement towards illness or death since this can be seen as a progressive, staged process.

Some proposals based on developmental theory are already well known to nurses. For example, Piaget (1932) clearly describes the stages through which he considers that a child progresses during development. He sees these stages as steps with fairly sudden transitions from one to another, rather than as a gentle slope. Thus at the initial sensori-motor stage, a child will only be aware of those things he can see or feel. The day will come when he will realize that objects suddenly hidden from sight are in fact still present but out of his view, and he will start to seek them out. He has reached the concrete stage. Ultimately he will progress to a third stage of formal operations where he can perceive distant objects accurately and understand their consistency. He has attained insight about the abstract world.

Other developmental theories identify concepts different from those of Piaget, but all are similar in that development is described as a series of stages, interspersed by visible transitions, rather than as a gradual unfolding. Each stage is superseded, in an orderly manner, by the next stage which may occur relatively promptly or over a more protracted period.

We also use the term development very widely in our everyday life: the development of a film, in a predictable staged direction; the failure to develop of a hyacinth bulb; the development of the signs and symptoms of an illness.

Five aspects of developmental models have been identified (Chin, 1980). They can be summarised as:

Direction This is the assumption that 'the system under observation is progressing somewhere'. As with systems theory, the thing which is under scrutiny may be very small, such as a cell or body organ; it may be a social system such as a community; it may be a psychological system such as an interpersonal relationship; or it may be the growth and development of people. It is assumed, however, that there is some implicit goal or end state that is being worked towards.

Identifiable states The most obvious examples of identifiable states in developmental theory are those described by Piaget. There are distinct characteristics which mark each stage, level or phase. An everyday example of stages would be the progress of frog spawn to tadpole and then the transition to a frog. Stages can also be seen in Maslow's hierarchy of needs (1954). According to his theory, higher level needs such as love, self-esteem and self-actualisation are only met when lower level ones such as physiological and safety needs have been met.

The movement from one identifiable state to another may be a sudden jump as of a child moving from primary to secondary school. Alternatively the transition may be more prolonged as in the metamorphosis from tadpole to frog. Clinically a changing state may occur suddenly, as it would following an unexpected bereavement, or more slowly, as it would in the episodic nature of a disease process such as multiple sclerosis.

Form of progression While change is inevitable, the course of the change may have certain characteristics. Four typical types of progression have been identified: linear, spiral, cyclical and branching.

A typical example of linear progression would be that of the movement from conception to death. It moves in one direction and unless there is an interruption, it will not regress.

Spiral progression can be seen when there is a return to the same subject at a higher level. This can be seen in the progress from simple sums to complex mathematics.

Cyclical progression is typically seen in problem-solving when the same system is applied to different situations.

Finally, branching progression is seen when there is a choice and the system can move in two or more directions. For instance, it may be the choice of occupation, the management of an illness or the selection of a partner for life. Branching progression also leads to more and more specialisation within an organisation. The point at

Linear Progress

Spiral Progress

Cyclical Progress

Branching Progress

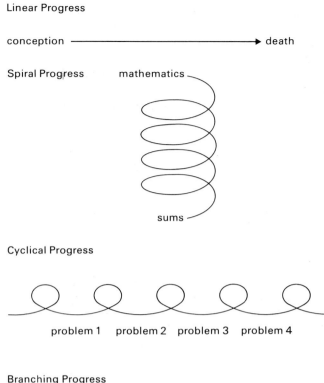

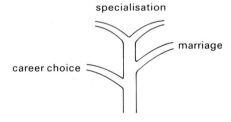

Fig. 3.2 *Forms of progression: linear, spiral, cyclical and branching.*

which a choice may be made can potentially lead to a developmental crisis.

Forces Forces are seen as the factors which lead to development. They have also been called stressors or stimuli and are the things which lead to change. There are many forces which lead to the development of people. These include hereditary factors, the environment, the interaction between the two, and the desire for self-actualisation. In day to day life we can sometimes recognise a particular force which has led to a change. It may be an individual who has inspired us, a trauma or disease, an alteration in social circumstances, or the acquisition of new knowledge. Alternatively the force may be less conspicuous, a maturation process inherent in all of us which may be triggered by some external factor.

Potentiality By potentiality it is meant that the conditions for growth and development, the 'potential', are built into the present state. Thus in Piaget's theory, the child has the potential to mature to adulthood. There is some variation in opinion about how much this potential is in fact influenced by surrounding circumstances.

While not all models use developmental theory as their major focus for construction, its influence can be seen in many of them. Peplau's (1952) model takes developmental theory as the major organising theme. Roper *et al.* (1980) give developmental theory less conspicuous attention but its presence can be felt. If part of nursing is seen as helping individuals to develop and grow, the application of developmental theory is obvious since it explains the direction and manner in which changes can occur.

Symbolic interaction

The essence of this theory is the interaction which occurs between people and their environment. The control does not lie with either one or the other, with either the person or his or her environment. Interaction theories focus on the relationships that people form with each other in their day to day lives, and on the way that relationships develop through a series of interactions. Rose (1980) lists some basic assumptions which underlie the symbolic interaction theory. They can be summarised as follows:

A person lives in a symbolic as well as a physical world In the physical world the individual receives stimuli through the senses of seeing, hearing, smelling, touching and tasting and will respond to these stimuli. However, over a period of time, the symbols which are perceived will take on particular values and meaning for the person. For example, the word or symbol 'ward' does not just mean the physical environment of beds, curtains, patients and staff. It may also mean caring and loving or pain and suffering. Thus, while in concrete terms the word 'ward' will have a similar meaning to most people, symbolically it may have many different meanings which have developed through previous interactions with other people in that environment and with that environment. The meaning of the word has resulted from the response of the one person to the symbol that has been received. Rose suggests that this ability is highly developed in human beings.

Through symbols people can evoke meanings and values other than their own in another person This assumption is associated with a person's ability to be aware of the values and meanings of others. It implies that one has empathy, can 'get under the skin' of others, and take on a particular role. In interaction of this kind where significant symbols are used, the communicator can only influence, rather than control the observer. Thus the process is social in nature, observers putting their own meanings and values

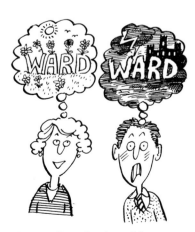

Fig. 3.3 *People view things differently.*

on the interaction. However, for the interaction to be meaningful, both participants must share similar meanings for words and movements. This raises issues about the many variations which occur in the use of both words and movements by people from different cultures and classes.

People learn symbolic meanings and values through interacting with others Each individual builds up an elaborate store of meanings and values through interaction with others. Similarly the way in which individuals interact will influence those around them. In time people can become skilled in knowing how others will react to them and adjust their behaviour accordingly. They can 'take on' specific roles in given situations which they have experienced previously in order to predict the responses.

Significant symbols usually occur in 'clusters' which dictate other values and meanings related to a cluster In this assumption it is suggested that there is a group of meanings and values which can be recognised by a particular society. It is linked with the idea of the way we interpret particular roles. There is a normally accepted pattern of behaviour by all members of a particular society in relationship to that role. For instance, the role of parent is linked with caring and providing for children. If a father deviates from that role and, for instance, rejects a child, it will affect his interaction with other people in the society in which he lives.

Davis (1975) describes the socialisation of nurses, where student nurses 'learn' to take on a pattern of behaviour acceptable to experienced nurses and often different from their original view, as an example of this process. It can also be seen in individuals who take on the 'patient role', which is seen to be acceptable to the hospital staff as they respond to the interactions with others in that setting.

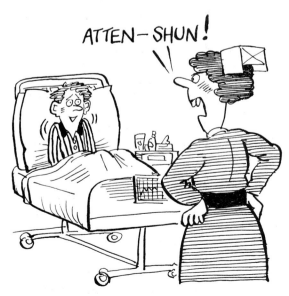

ATTEN–SHUN!

Fig. 3.4 *People often adopt the role of the patient.*

Most people have a number of roles which they take on according to the group of people with whom they are interacting at a given time. They usually accept symbols for each of these roles according to the society in which they live. They will, however, also have a 'whole person' role which is linked with the value and meaning they place on themselves as individuals.

It is possible to assess future courses of action through a thinking process rather than resorting to behaviour based on trial and error
Since the logical conclusion of the process of symbolic interaction is that responses to a given situation can be predicted, trial and error behaviour is unnecessary. The way an individual predicts the future is based on his past and present experience. It also influences his present interaction. His ability for symbolic interaction heightens his awareness of the values and meanings of others.

While this theory may sound complex on first reading, its relevance to nursing is undeniable. Empathy, a quality inherent in symbolic interaction, is a characteristic often cited as essential to nursing. Similarly an understanding of the variety of roles we all play and the way in which they have developed can only help to enhance nursing. Threads of this theory are seen in most models. For instance Roy talks about self-concept and interdependence as important areas of assessment. Symbolic interaction is the major focus of King's model (1971).

As we have already said, there is an element of all these theories in most models of nursing. We recognise that they do not make for easy reading but hope that we have been able to represent them in relatively simple terms without losing too much of their essence.

Models based on these theories all, however, seem to agree on a number of concepts about patients and nursing. The most important of these concepts are:

- Health.
- The holistic view of people.
- The humanistic view of people.
- The autonomy of patients and clients.
- The need to develop a productive or therapeutic relationship between those who nurse, and those who are nursed.

Human nature

It has already been suggested that the basis of the practice of any service-orientated group lies in the beliefs and values that are held by that group. In outlining the biomedical model of practice on which most health care has been based until recent times, the dualistic approach — the division of mind and body — proposed by René Descartes was described. The result of such an approach has been an enormous increase in both knowledge and skills. However, over the last century other views of people have emerged which are now starting to influence our thoughts about the way in which nurses practise. The two most influential ones are those of *holism* and *humanism*. They are common features of the majority of models of nursing which will be described in this book and therefore they warrant further discussion.

Holism

The word 'holism' was first introduced by Jan Christian Smuts (1926), a South African philosopher in the early part of this century. Holism relates to the study of the whole organism or of whole systems, its spelling arising from the Greek word 'holos'. (The English spelling with a 'w' is a relatively recent fourteenth century innovation!)

Underlying a holistic view of people are two basic assumptions or beliefs:

1. The individual always responds as a unified whole.

2. Individuals as a whole are different from and more than the sum of their parts.

Both these assumptions mean that there is now movement away from the ideas proposed by Descartes who claimed that, in order to study the body as a machine, it could be broken down into its component parts. If the assumptions of holism are accepted, it indicates that there is a need to study the whole being, and the manner in which the body and mind interact.

Byrne and Thompson (1978) use the analogy of water to describe this phenomenon. Water as a whole is made up of two components, namely hydrogen and oxygen. Similarly when considering people there are at least two major components, namely the body and the mind; some people may choose to include a third spiritual component. If the properties of the components of water are considered separately, they each have distinct characteristics. Oxygen will support combustion. Hydrogen is potentially explosive. However, when they are put together in the particular combination that makes water, a completely different property, that of extinguishing fire, arises. Thus the whole is different from the sum of the parts. If the parts are studied independently rather than in unity, an inaccurate picture of water will emerge.

The underlying belief in a holistic view of people follows a similar view. By considering the functioning of the body without taking into consideration the response of the mind and spirit, an inaccurate picture of that person will emerge. Such inaccuracy will lead to difficulty in helping people solve problems and hence, in the long run, lead to extra cost both in terms of human suffering and money.

This view is not entirely unsupported by scientific evidence. As a young medical student, Hans Selye observed what he later described as a 'syndrome of just being sick' (1978). Unable in his early medical career to distinguish between the specific signs or symptoms of many diseases, he was aware of the similarities in many cases. Much later he was to reconsider this early observation and, through a series of experiments, conclude that there was in fact a syndrome, the general adaptation syndrome (GAS) occurring in the body when it was exposed to stress, whether the stress was physical or psychological in origin. Pietroni (1984) describes Selye as the 'father of modern stress work' and acknowledges his contribution in 'the difficult and painstaking job of putting body and mind back together again'. Selye's influence can also be seen quite clearly in many of the models of nursing described. The importance of stress, as an influence in development as well as a cause of ill health when occurring in excess, is recognised in many models. Since the word 'stress' has become so widely used both professionally and by lay people, there are variations in its interpretation; some people only think of the physical side and others only consider psychological factors. Furthermore, it is often only considered in a negative manner as something that is harmful, whereas in fact it is also the stimulus for development and growth. The notion of stress is a common feature of many models, although it is not always referred to by the actual word 'stress'.

Humanism

The second underlying value which can frequently be recognised in nursing models is that of humanism. Humanism is often linked with a second school of thought known as existentialism.

Humanism is based on the value of being human, of existing and of the quality of that existence. It places great emphasis on the nature of people. The emphasis of existentialism is also on people but stresses the individual human being. Stevenson (1974) describes three main characteristics of existentialism. The first is the uniqueness of the individual person. He suggests that general theories about people are secondary to the importance of the individual. The second part is related to the 'meaning and purpose of human lives rather than . . . truths about the whole universe and how it works'. The third point that Stevenson makes, and maybe the one which is most relevant to us, is the freedom of individuals to choose. This is seen as the most valued human characteristic. Thus there is freedom for an individual to direct his own life, choose his own attitudes and behaviours.

The principles of humanistic existentialism have been subsumed by both Christian and atheist philosophers. For instance, Stevenson describes the view suggested by Kierkegaard that there are three main ways of life between which an individual could choose. These were the aesthetic way concerned with beauty, the ethical way concerned with ethical questions and the religious way relating to God's direction and will. In Kierkegaard's view the religious way of life was the highest choice that an individual could make but he suggested that 'it can only be reached by a free leap into the arms of God'.

Alternatively J. P. Sartre was an existentialist atheist, denying the existence of God. In his opinion humans are condemned to be free. We have no choice but to be free and cannot blame the course of our lives on the will of a higher being. Such freedom is, in his view, not a happy state. He feels we are responsible for our emotions and reactions. Thus, a statement such as 'I am stupid' is not to assert a fact already in existence, since we control what we make of our lives ourselves, but to anticipate how society will react to the resulting behaviour. We have the choice ourselves of changing the behaviour which leads us to attribute such characteristics to ourselves.

Bevis (1978) sees humanistic existentialism as the 'natural maturational philosophy for nursing'. Indeed, within the philosophy of humanistic existentialism are many of the ideas which are being discussed by nurses today, such as the value of human beings, their uniqueness as individuals, the quality of life and the freedom to choose — all topical subjects that are now widely debated within nursing. The application of humanism to health care would suggest that individuals should be able to make choices about how their health is managed and to explore methods which are complementary to either traditional medicine or traditional nursing. It also emphasises the responsibility of the individual in such circumstances.

Holism and humanism are not only reflected in many of the nursing models, they can also be recognised in society's changing attitudes to health and medicine. For example, there is an upsurge of interest in holistic medicine. Community Health Councils and Patients' Associations have been established. Doctors are being publicly challenged about the right to control and direct all health care by both patients and other health care workers alike. As Bevis says — 'The current philosophy that is swaying nursing thought and action is humanistic existentialism'.

Patient/client autonomy

Characteristic of most nursing models is the belief that the clients or patients are individuals who have the right to be involved in making informed choices about themselves and their future. This belief is often referred to as 'patient autonomy', and autonomy is defined as the freedom to make decisions within the limits of competence of the individual; the opposite of autonomy is having to comply with dictates from people who are in a superior position. The belief of autonomy suggests that we value patients and their contribution to their own health care.

Some models give more emphasis to the concept of autonomy than others. The model described by Orem (1980), which focuses on self-care, gives considerable emphasis to autonomy. As expounded in Orem's model, self-care is a good example of the notion of autonomy applied to a model for practice, and may serve to demonstrate its implications. Levin *et al*. (1979) define self-care as 'a process whereby a lay person functions on his/her own behalf in health promotion and prevention, and in disease detection and

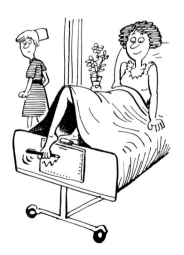

Fig. 3.5 *Patient autonomy.*

treatment'. It therefore relies on the belief that the person who is the subject of nursing has both the ability and the right to be involved in choosing what happens to him or her. This belief arose from health care consumers, customers or patients in the 1960s, and began with anti-professional and anti-intellectual feelings which were popular at the time. There was a general desire by many people to return to a way of life which emphasised humanity, respect and sharing. This can be seen as a reaction to materialism and mechanistic practices in the world as a whole, as well as in the practice of nurses and other health workers. Health workers and 'professional people' in other disciplines still pursue practice which views the client as being dependent on them and therefore needing to be placed in a role whereby they seek help and are told what to do. Many nursing models concentrate on perceiving people's individual identities and rights and are therefore moving away from practice which directs people towards practice which supports and enables them to learn and use this learning to make their own decisions. Illich (1975) describes how increased professionalism in health care, and therefore a focus on a view of the patient which places him in a position inferior to the practitioner, have led to the point where significant levels of human suffering are the very result of the professional practice of medicine, something he calls 'iatrogenesis'. He says that:

> 'once society is so organised that medicine can transform people into patients because they are unborn, newborn, menopausal or some other "at risk age" the population inevitably loses some of its autonomy to its healers.'

Many other writers on health care stress how the professional worker can effectively remove the individual's right to autonomous decision-making for highly tenuous reasons, and that professional power can be exerted to make clients comply with professional values.

The belief in patient/client autonomy inherent in many nursing models assumes that, if responsibility for healthy living and health care is vested in the individual concerned and not a professional, health and recovery is more likely to occur. All patients should have the freedom to identify their own needs, and to decide on how these needs should be met. In practical terms for example, the sick people being cared for by nurses should be given the power to make their own decisions about how they will be nursed. This may entail either selecting particular ways of carrying out a daily living activity or choosing to give the responsibility for the decisions to the nurse, because they feel unwell and are unable to decide for themselves. This latter option is an important one to stress because autonomy for patients does not necessarily mean that they *must* constantly make decisions — it simply means that they have enough power to choose whether to decide for themselves or to allow others to decide for them. Such a belief gives rise to another major concept which underlies many nursing models — that of the central importance of the relationship between helper and helped — the nurse and the patient.

Partnership in the nurse/patient relationship

In models where the autonomy of the individual client is recognised, the practice of the discipline, its goals, and the knowledge needed to achieve them, are fundamentally different from those where the model focuses on a client who needs the expert intervention of the practitioner. The practitioner operates as a partner in practice *with* the client rather than a director of practice *to*, *for*, or *at* the client. In order to do this the practitioner has to share what he or she knows with the patient, rather than withholding this knowledge and telling the patient what is best. In this way patients become as knowledgeable about the various options which can be chosen to overcome their specific problems and are able to make their own choices. Partnership also demands that the practitioner complements the patient's own uniqueness and adapts knowledge to the patient's abilities and needs and passes it on so that both can work out a plan of action instead of the practioner 'plying a trade' on a take-it-or-leave-it basis.

In nursing, developing a relationship with a patient based on partnership conflicts with the popular biomedical model and assumes a different role for nurses and a different knowledge base. It suggests that the individual who needs nursing actually needs a practitioner who establishes a close relationship based on equality, and it emphasises patient teaching to enable individuals to make informed choices. The majority of nursing models advocate partnership, and therefore the ability to teach, motivate and communicate and an understanding of psychology and sociology are included in the skills and knowledge that nurses need in order to nurse according to these models.

Traditional practice based on the biomedical model concentrates on telling patients what to do. Health care workers ask the patients 'would you like to. . . ?', but they expect compliance. Non-compliance is not approved of and sometimes sanctions are applied. For example, the elderly obese lady who needs to lose weight if the soreness under her breast is to subside, may be forced to eat non-fattening food even if she would prefer to tolerate the sore skin rather than the longing she feels for food when she is forced to diet. Although the values held by nurses may mean that they see dieting as the only choice, partnership demands that the elderly lady should be made fully aware, through teaching, of the value of losing weight. However, on the basis of partnership she should still have the power to choose to eat fattening foods without the nurse showing disapproval or applying sanctions.

All of these issues, which relate to patients or clients, are represented to a greater or lesser degree in the majority of nursing models. All models also express views on nursing and the nurse, and the common characteristics associated with these are considered in the next chapter.

4

Common Characteristics of Nursing Models — The Nurse and Nursing

The issues that have been discussed in Chapter 3 have been mainly related to patients themselves. Those discussed in this chapter concern patients, nurses and how nursing takes place. They include: views on health; views on nurses as part of the health care team; and accountability for nursing practice.

Health as the focus of nursing

All models for health care workers include views about what health is, with the biomedical model viewing health as the absence of disease or disorder. Nursing models on the whole perceive health as a much wider concept relating to wellness and the achievement of potential, but, like the biomedical model, they see the goal of practice revolving round the achievement of this thing called health.

The biomedical model view of health or wellness is based on the concept of physiological homeostasis. The World Health Organisation (1948) definition broadened the biomedical view of health out to 'a state of complete physical, mental and social well-being and not merely the absence of disease or infirmity'. This can be loosely seen to mean physiological, psychological and sociological homeostasis. Both of these biomedical views — the more restricted one and the broader one — have been criticised. In particular, the definition of the WHO is said to be utopian and its very broadness may mean that few people, if any, can be considered healthy. It proposes a static state of complete well-being and opposes ideas about the dynamic nature of healthiness. Furthermore, many people, particularly medical sociologists, argue that the absence of disease is not an accurate description of the healthy state.

To be fair to those who currently practise according to the supposedly 'objective' biomedical model, the physiological concept of homeostasis is often expanded beyond the realms of biology and may encompass:

- Body balance.
- Psychological and emotional balance.

- Cultural, social and political balance.
- Spiritual and philosophical balance.

Nevertheless, the biomedical model sees disease, no matter how it defines the term, as something which can be resolved by the application of scientific knowledge, thus applying science as a means to achieve a state of health.

Some people see health as a different concept from wellness, while others suggest that both terms are interchangeable. It seems appropriate to us to agree with the latter view. Both wellness and health are frequently explained by either/or propositions — that is, one is either ill or well, diseased or healthy. In order for people to know that they are ill, they must have some concept of what is 'normal' against which to measure their current physical or mental condition. Those who support a rigid biomedical model regard illness as a deviation from a biological norm and health or wellness as the maintenance of homeostasis in a physiological sense.

This view does not answer an important question: is health or wellness an objective state which is defined by doctors? Or, is it a subjective state perceived by individuals about themselves and influenced by what the community they live in think about what is normal?

Wellness and illness are universal phenomena. Everybody, everywhere has ideas about what 'being healthy' is. However, there is no universal definition. What is health or wellness differs markedly between groups. For example, in Western society scabies is seen as unacceptable and unhealthy, whereas because of its endemic nature in some Third World countries and the limited treatment provisions

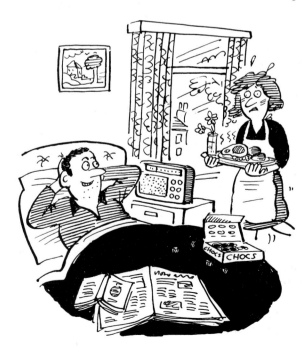

Fig. 4.1 *The sick role carries privileges (for some!).*

available, it is seen there as merely an irritating fact of life. Sociological theorists see illness as a deviation from social norms, that is something which is not regarded as a normal way of social living. Health and illness are therefore related to problems of deviance, conformity and social control. Friedson (1975) sees this social deviance as conduct which violates sufficiently valued norms. In concrete terms, this may mean lying in bed all day and being unable to do normal everyday things like shopping, talking and keeping clean and tidy.

In communities where being independent in these activities is normal, this sort of behaviour would be a deviance, a behaviour which is seen as abnormal. Most sociologists tend to define what is *not* health or wellness in order to then describe what it is. Parsons (1951) however defined health as 'the state of optimum capacity for effective performance of valued tasks'. In effect, therefore, a person is well if he or she is able to conform to society's views of what is normal in terms of behaviour and carrying out certain tasks. The person who behaves in a way which society approves of, works in such a way and plays in such a way, can be regarded as being healthy and well. On the other hand, the person who shouts obscenities to people who wear red hats, or who is unable to get on and off the bus without help, may be seen in some societies (certainly our own) as being unwell or ill.

Field (1972) has put forward yet another view; he differentiates between illness and disease. Illness is, he says, the person's subjective experience of ill health, whereas disease is the medical conception of pathological abnormality. Figure 4.2 shows a schema to describe the relationship between disease and illness.

Following this schema, illness may be present or absent in disease, and people may feel ill even if there is no evidence of disease.

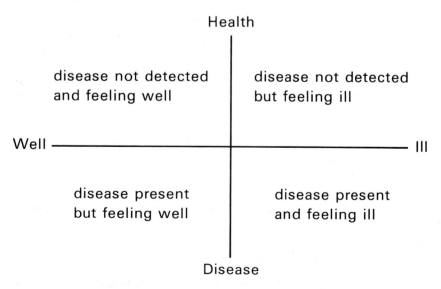

Fig. 4.2 *Perceptions of health, disease, wellness and illness.*

This idea of disease and illness suggests therefore that health is merely the opposite of disease and wellness the opposite of illness.

Many nursing models consider that nursing should concern itself with wellness and health. If we agree with Field's view, we could therefore suggest that nursing exists to serve not only those who are said to be ill by medical diagnosis but also those who *feel* ill. If, on the other hand, we see health as the state in which people function well enough to conform with what is expected of them from the community they live in, then it is obvious that 'health' will vary from society to society. What is considered to be well in a poor region of South America may be very different from that of an affluent area of London. For example, the presence of minor aches in the back may be regarded as a perfectly natural, normal state in the former but may be seen as a reason for a prosperous Londoner to take to his or her bed.

Illness has to be legitimised or seen as valid by the societal group we live in before the position of being well and healthy ceases to exist. If the society sees a runny nose and headaches as being merely minor irritations, the person with a common cold will still be regarded as being relatively healthy and will not be allowed to be regarded as a sick person. The concept of health is therefore determined in the sociological view by the society. Those of us who live in Western society may, according to Parsons, be ascribed a sick role when we feel ill by the non-sick others. If this happens, certain privileges are given, but we have to fulfil certain obligations. The privileges are such things as being allowed to stay in bed, to stay off work and to have things done for us. The obligations are such things as having to have the sick role legitimised or made acceptable by a doctor stating a specific diagnosis. Neither are we allowed to do things which appear to be healthy. For example, looking ill and being able to say that the doctor said you had influenza may give you the privileges of time off from work and of having breakfast brought to bed. But if you jog around the park, go to the pub or disco or dig in the garden, you would not be meeting the obligations of the sick role and therefore the privileges may be withdrawn.

The values of society influence lay perceptions of illness and health. Apple (1960) describes two criteria by which people in Western society judge themselves to be ill:

1. The recency and novelty of the experience (when it has just happened and hasn't happened before).

2. The degree to which it interferes with ordinary activities.

To judge wellness, Bauman (1961) says that we use three criteria:

1. The subjective feeling of well-being.

2. The absence of any symptoms.

3. Being able to perform activities which those in good health can perform.

The sociological view of health sees illness as a form of deviance, determined by society itself, and certain rules or criteria seem to exist in each society to enable this to occur. Health or wellness is based on being able to behave in certain ways and carry out the tasks which are expected for a person to conform with what is seen as 'normal'. Health care systems, and therefore nursing, are seen as mechanisms of social control to ensure isolation and treatment of ill members of society.

Both the biomedical and sociological views of health and wellness are relevant to the discussion on health as a focus of nursing, but in isolation they do not match up to the common features of nursing models.

Nursing theorists attempt in many models to outline health or wellness from a holistic stance, which incorporates social and biological views, but includes other concepts. They frequently emphasise the 'reaching of potential' as the central concept in defining health. Rogers (1970) says that wellness is a feeling of wholeness and uniqueness. She describes it as:

1. 'A state of homeo-dynamic balance of energy.'

2. 'A continually evolving of direction of growth.'

3. 'A sense of predictability, pattern and organisation of life.'

4. 'A sense of satisfaction with one's ability to conceptualize, think, imagine, communicate and experience sensations and feelings.'

Such sentiments and beliefs, although rather poetic, are common to practically all models for nursing practice. They come from the current linking of nursing to the beliefs in such things as holism, humanistic existentialism and the right to autonomy which have been emphasised in this book. How we think about health is of course determined by our beliefs about human nature and, since nursing increasingly sees the human race as being made up of individuals who must be regarded in a whole way, the belief that health must be regarded holistically and from the perspective of the individual concerned is a logical basis for practice. The goals of models for nursing practice all, in some way, relate to the achievement of health, and health is almost always seen as the individual achieving his or her maximum potential. This incorporates the concepts of biological, sociological, psychological and spiritual balance or homeostasis. The knowledge and skill base required in nursing models includes those which will enable the nurse to promote health in individuals.

Nursing in relation to the multidisciplinary clinical team

'The term multi-disciplinary team is used to describe the group of National Health Service and other workers who are contributing to a patient's (or client's) health or care.' So says the secretariat of the Royal Commission on the National Health Service (1978). A whole range of disciplines work together to provide health care including physiotherapists, occupational therapists, doctors, dietitians, domestics, nursing auxiliaries, porters and many more. All, of course, hold a model to picture their work and the work of others. Health care workers by their very definition all broadly aim for health or wellness of the client, but each occupational and professional group will hold different perspectives on specific aspects of the nature of people and will have particular goals which are different from other groups. They will therefore require different knowledge, skills, and attitudes.

Because of their common interest in the promotion of health, most of them will share common beliefs as well as beliefs specific to their discipline. For example, nurses, physiotherapists and occupational therapists may all see independence in daily living as a right of the client and would include that as one of the goals of practice. Similarly, all three would acknowledge a need for knowledge of anatomy and physiology, skills in patient teaching and motivation, and attitudes which include valuing the patient as an individual. Each, however, would have a different focus within these areas. A model for physiotherapy practice may focus on independence in body movement and on knowledge of the anatomy and physiology of muscles and soft tissues.

Alternatively the occupational therapist may place more emphasis on specific and complete acts of living such as cooking or washing up and may concentrate more on being knowledgeable about fine movements and the design of aids to support daily living acts than the physiotherapist. Nursing, too, has a different focus. If it didn't, then why have nurses at all? Although models for practice of all health workers are bound to overlap and share many similarities, the whole basis of multidisciplinary team work is the bringing together of people who are able to practise from different model bases acquired through professional training.

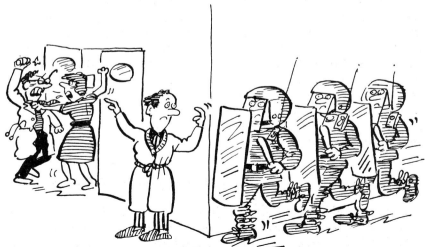

Fig. 4.3 *Without explicit models for practice, conflict can occur.*

This may sound like 'common sense' and hardly worthy of much discussion. For multidisciplinary teams to work together, however, it is absolutely vital that each other's role and basis for practice is understood and accepted by each discipline. Each member of the team can justify membership only if he or she has something to contribute that cannot be done as well by other members of the team.

Although a major function of nurses is to coordinate the contributions of the team members (because nurses, and nurses alone, provide a service which spans 24 hours in both hospitals and the community), there must be some specific contributions to patient care which are clearly 'nursing' if nurses are needed at all. The development of models to describe nursing's contribution to patient care is therefore essential if patients are to receive a service which is acceptable. Such a service can only be achieved if the teamwork it requires is unmarred by conflict between members or individual people working in isolation. This can arise if the different disciplines are unable to be clear about what they believe in, aim for, and know about. Therefore cooperation will only be possible if these disciplines can offer such a picture of their practice to each other. Nursing has been particularly disadvantaged in playing a full part in team work because of its inability or reluctance to be clear about its contribution. The need to be clear increases as time progresses because of the acceleration of specialisation in health care which we discussed earlier in relationship to the reductionist approach being valued in Western society. Nursing teams are members of a much bigger multidisciplinary clinical team, but their contribution to care can, and must, be equal to that of the contributions of others. Sometimes the contribution of a specific discipline will inevitably be greater because of the needs of the patient, but this will change as the patient's needs change. For example, the elderly gentleman with a severe headache with an obvious physiological cause and resolvable by taking a certain drug will clearly need the contribution of the medical member of the multidisciplinary clinical team in primary health care and will need very little from other members. However, if the headache makes him dizzy and unable to meet his daily living needs, the district nurse may have to contribute just as much to his care as, and sometimes far more than, the general practitioner.

There is much argument about the nature of the multidisciplinary team work between disciplines, particularly in relation to leadership. Many doctors argue that they have the greatest contribution to make to care and therefore should always lead the other health care disciplines. On the other hand, some nurses dispute this and suggest that leadership should be determined for each individual patient on the basis of which professional worker is best suited to lead the care. Many nurses who have started looking at nursing from the basis of a model for practice consider that some patients primarily need medical care with the help of others — so the doctor should lead the care: some primarily need physiotherapy with the help of others — so the physiotherapist should lead the care; and some primarily need nursing with the help of others — so the nurse should lead the care. Such a view could, they argue, be applied to all professional health care workers, and McFarlane (1978) says:

> ... it is no longer appropriate that doctors should assume primacy over other professions, taking the major responsibility for care. I suggest that medical leadership of the team often restricts the full assessment of health needs, particularly in cases where the medical model of care is inappropriate to the problem, e.g. in terminal care.

It is not possible, in this discussion, to consider the argument about the nature of multidisciplinary teams in depth, because the background is complex and would need a book in itself. However, it is clear that only a limited contribution can be made until nurses in any team are able to describe their particular contribution with clarity. Agreeing on a model for practice is an important and essential beginning to multidisciplinary clinical team work in health care.

Accountability for practice

There is a great deal of discussion at the moment about whether or not nurses can, or should, be held accountable for their own practice. The answer to such a question is the single most important factor in the development of nursing. If nurses are not prepared as an occupational group to stand accountable for their own decision-making and actions, then they cannot expect either patients or other colleagues working in health care to value or respect their opinions.

So what is this thing called 'accountability' and how does it relate to models for practice? According to Lewis and Batey (1982) accountability implies 'formal obligation to disclose'. You must be able to say:

1. What it is you are trying to achieve (your goal).

2. How you are trying to achieve it (your actions).

3. The justification for your actions (your knowledge base).

4. The outcome of your actions (your evaluation).

In other words nursing actions must be explainable, defendable and based on knowledge rather than tradition or myth. We have found it a salutary exercise to ask ourselves whether we are in a position to respond accurately to some of the questions posed above. Without a clear statement of intent, it is impossible to justify why certain actions have been taken. Without evaluation, it is impossible to know whether or not our actions have been effective in helping a patient or client to either maintain or move towards his or her desired goal. Many nursing actions today are based on traditional myths, for instance the routine observations carried out in so many circumstances which can be both time consuming for nurses and disruptive for the patient. Why are they being taken? What are the criteria on which a decision is made for them to start or stop? Another commonly given example of a nursing tradition is the addition of salt to the bath. When there is no evidence of its therapeutic effect, how can there be justification for continuing a practice which is largely based on folklore?

We (1984) suggest that there are two major criteria which have to be met in order for a nurse to be accountable. First, there must be a statement about the expected outcome or the goal which it is hoped will be achieved. Second, there must be an established system of evaluation in order to see whether or not this goal has been achieved.

One of the functions of a model of nursing is to identify the broad goal of practice, although it may be as broad or as unspecific as to cure disease or to strive towards self-care and independence. Once this broad philosophically-based goal has been agreed upon within a team, it becomes much easier to identify goals in day to day practice. Not only will it give guidance to the identification of goals, but also to the part to be played by all concerned. A very simple example is the difference in action of two nurses working with a patient with a colostomy. One will attend to the colostomy for the patient, perhaps with a goal of keeping the patient clean. The second will assist the patient in caring for his or her own colostomy, possibly in this case with a goal based on the belief in self-care or

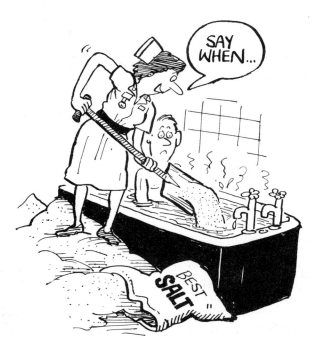

Fig. 4.4 *Some practice is based on folklore.*

independence. If these two nurses are working in the same area, the result for the patient can only be confusion. However, if the team of nurses agrees upon the model of nursing on which they base their practice such confusion can be avoided.

Accountability and responsibility

There is a considerable lack of clarity about the two notions of accountability and responsibility, different authorities interpreting them in different ways. Some people use the words interchangeably, while others clearly differentiate between them. Because it is unclear, it is important to try to clarify these issues.

While the two ideas are inextricably linked, there is a clear difference between them. Accountability implies that a situation has been assessed, a plan has been made and carried out, and the results evaluated. Responsibility refers to the task or 'charge'. Thus nurses can be offered the 'charge' or responsibility for carrying out a particular action. In agreeing to accept the responsibility for that action, they become accountable for fulfilling it.

A job description usually itemises the 'tasks' for which an individual is responsible. In agreeing to fulfil that job description, the individual becomes accountable for carrying them out. In this instance, the body to whom he or she is accountable will be the employing authority. However, at a clinical level, the agreement will be that the nurse will accept the responsibility for delivering nursing care. It becomes obvious then, that the nurse must be accountable to the recipient of the service that is offered, that is the patient or client. This line of accountability, between the giver of care or the nurse and the recipient of care or the patient, is the most important one. Nurses must be in a position to explain and defend their actions either to the patients or the bodies which protect patients.

The major function of the United Kingdom Central Council (UKCC) and the National Boards is to protect patients. These bodies were established in response to an Act of Parliament, its remit being to ensure that safe standards of practice are offered by nurses. In order to achieve this aim, they have to establish the criteria which they recognise as the minimal level of achievement which an individual must attain in order to be called a nurse. In other words they must be able to identify what nursing is, the purpose of nursing or the goals it is trying to achieve, and the knowledge and skills that are necessary to achieve these goals. Without this background, they would not be able to fulfil their function of protecting the public.

The National Boards have been given the 'charge' or responsibility of approving the educational programmes for nurses. A review of earlier syllabi which were established by their predecessor, the General Nursing Council for England and Wales, demonstrates that these syllabi were largely based on the biomedical model already described. However, this emphasis is now changing, evidenced by the most recently produced syllabus for Registered Mental Handicap Nurses (1982). It is based on three guiding principles, namely:

- 'People with mental handicap have the same rights and, as far as possible, the same responsibilities as other members of the community.

- People with mental handicap have a right and a need to live like others in the community and to receive services that meet their changing needs.

- People with mental handicap should receive additional help from professional services to allow the full recognition and expression of their individuality.'

With these principles in mind the syllabus concentrates on developing an individual nurse's skill in order to practise as an advocate and a teacher as well as to deliver the traditional nurturing care of nursing. The resulting course for nursing students emphasises helping the student to:

> . . . . develop insight into his/her own needs as a person so that they may develop relationships with people with mental handicap as valued individuals.

Ideally it could be argued that a single unified model of nursing should be agreed upon in order to bring uniformity into practice. However, we feel very strongly that clinical nurses should have the right to choose the detailed model on which they base their practice. Nevertheless the influence of the value systems, the goals of practice, and the knowledge and skills required are reflected within a syllabus. This is one way in which the central controlling bodies of nursing can demonstrate to the public their accountability for protecting patients.

Use of an explicit model for practice is an essential beginning to accountability and responsibility in nursing. It will clarify what nursing is, helping individual practitioners to decide what work they will agree to accept. It will identify for all nurses the knowledge they require to practice. In day to day work the model will be the guiding force which will help them to decide what to assess, how to plan and set goals, what part they will take in the action and what to evaluate.

Existing nursing models

Having explored the 'hard core' of nursing models in these first four chapters, we can now look at specific models described by nurses for nurses in the literature. In the next six chapters, we describe specific models for practice, using the structure already introduced, of:

1. The beliefs and values on which the model is based.

2. The goals of nursing practice.

3. The knowledge and skills the nurse needs to develop in order to achieve these goals.

In order to show how they may be applied practically, each chapter also includes an assessment framework and a brief care plan derived from the model described. They are not intended to be 'ideal' examples but are merely used to demonstrate how each model can be used in practice.

We have deliberately limited these following chapters to an account of the specific concepts of each model on the assumption that the common issues already discussed in earlier chapters will be linked to them.

Relating nursing models to the assessment phase of the nursing process

The nursing process is currently seen as an effective way of delivering nursing — a method of carrying it through. But the nursing itself has to be made clear through agreeing on a model. One model may be selected; an amalgamation of a number of them; or a framework developed by the nursing team itself.

The 'process' cannot happen without an agreement on 'nursing'. The most concrete example of how a model affects practice is the structure it gives to assessment. For example, the biomedical model sees the patient as being made up of body systems, and those who practise according to this model would logically structure assessment according to these systems. Some doctors use a structured assessment form reflecting this belief, which would follow the outline below:

Complains of:
History of present condition:
Past medical history:
Social history:
Functional enquiry:
Drugs:
Allergies:
O/E Central nervous system:
    Respiratory system:
    etc.

This is obviously based on body systems and on the goal of practice being related to the diagnosis and treatment of disease or illness.

Specific nursing models give clear direction to the structure of the nursing assessment as well as to identifying patient problems amenable to nursing actions, to goal setting, to care planning, to implementation and to evaluation. To demonstrate this practical application of each model, an assessment of a patient, based on the model under discussion, is included in each chapter.

Some of the nursing models we describe may 'ring a bell' immediately and mean something to you personally and to the sort of practice you are currently engaged in. Others may have less meaning for you or be less relevant to your interest. All of them, however, are serious attempts by nurses to use concepts and theories to represent the reality of nursing practice.

Throughout the following six chapters we describe some aspects of nursing for one specific patient and show how the approaches to care vary according to the model. While there are similarities in the basic difficulty identified as being experienced by the patient, the approach, recording, goal setting and management are all slightly different and are dependent on the specific beliefs and goals of the model.

The patient concerned is Mr Gordon Smith, a 67 year old man who has had rheumatoid arthritis since the age of 46 years. The onset of the disease occurred two years after his wife's death but he has lived alone ever since this time, valuing his independence and ability to run his own home. Recently his physical condition has deteriorated and he has been admitted to hospital for review of his treatment by the rheumatologist.

One of Mr Smith's problems relates to an inadequate dietary intake and consideration of this specific problem will be pursued from the different perspectives of each model described. An assessment of his needs is given in each case, followed by problem identification, goal setting, planning of action (showing the involvement of both the nurse and the patient), and evaluation. We hope that this will allow a comparison of the various models for nursing and help individual readers to consider which model is closest to his or her own views of nursing.

5

The Activities of Living Model for Nursing

The 'Activities of Living' model was developed by Nancy Roper, Winifred Logan and Alison Tierney (Roper, Logan and Tierney, 1980) and arose from the findings of a research project on the clinical experience of student nurses (Roper, 1976). This model was the first attempt by British nurses to develop a conceptual model for nursing, and it has become widely used in the United Kingdom, especially by nurse educators in developing curricula.

Many nurses see the activities of living model as a modification of Virginia Henderson's concept of nursing, which has been internationally accepted as an authoritative definition of the nature of nursing (Henderson, 1966).

Although the activities of living model incorporates most of the issues discussed in the first four chapters, such as holism, partnership and health, its essence is the idea that all individuals are involved in activities which enable them to live and grow.

Living activities

Perhaps the most widely known definition of nursing is that of Virginia Henderson (1966):

> The unique function of the nurse is to assist the individual, sick or well, in the performance of those activities contributing to health or its recovery (or to a peaceful death) that he would perform unaided if he had the necessary strength, will or knowledge, and to do this in such a way as to help him to gain independence as rapidly as possible.

She goes on to describe what nursing does by listing 14 'activities of daily living'. She suggests that nursing is:

'Helping the patient with the following activities or providing conditions under which he can perform them unaided:

1. Breathe normally.

2. Eat and drink adequately.

3. Eliminate body wastes.

4. Move and maintain desirable postures.

5. Sleep and rest.

6. Select suitable clothes — dress and undress.

7. Maintain body temperature within normal range by adjusting clothing and modifying the environment.

8. Keep the body clean and well groomed and protect the integument (i.e. *the skin*).

9. Avoid dangers in the environment and avoid injuring others.

10. Communicate with others in expressing emotions, needs, fears or opinions.

11. Worship according to one's faith.

12. Work in such a way that there is a sense of accomplishment.

13. Play or participate in various forms of recreation.

14. Learn, discover, or satisfy the curiosity that leads to normal development and health, and use the available health facilities.'

This approach to analysing nursing has become well accepted by British nurses, and Roper, Logan and Tierney have developed Henderson's concept into a model which focuses on the activities people engage in to live.

Beliefs and values

This model focuses on the client as an individual engaged in living throughout his or her lifespan, and moving from dependence to independence, according to age, circumstances and environment. The important ideas underlying the model are therefore: the progression along a lifespan; a dependence/independence continuum; and the activities of living.

Life span An individual is seen to begin living at conception, and to end it at death — a somewhat obvious fact perhaps, but an important part of the model. As people engage in the process of living, their position on the life span influences their capacity for independence.

The dependence/independence continuum This is moved along dynamically and is affected by a whole range of factors. For example, newborn babies will be at the dependent end of the continuum because they are not mature enough to be independent in many activities of living. Mature adults of 30 years may be at the independent end in virtually all of the activities of living, but may become dependent if illness or trauma occurs or if they are placed in an environment with which they are unfamiliar, for example, the middle of the Amazon jungle.

The activities of living The model sees individuals as engaging in 12 basic activities of living. However, there are stages in the lifespan when the individual cannot yet, or no longer can, perform one or more of the activities. Specific circumstances may also restrict performance in one or more of the activities.

The twelve activities are:

- Maintaining a safe environment
- Breathing
- Eliminating
- Controlling body temperature
- Working and playing
- Sleeping
- Communicating
- Eating and drinking
- Personal cleansing and dressing
- Mobilising
- Expressing sexuality
- Dying

Each activity is seen to have 3 components — physical or physiological, social and psychological. For example, eating involves the passage of nutrients through various anatomical structures and being acted upon by various physiological processes. The nutrients themselves have a chemical basis and physiological purpose. Eating and nutrition is also affected by psychological factors, with some people eating to meet psychological needs and others not eating because of psychological influences. Eating is also a social act: for example, in Western society, people may eat fruit cake at a wedding because it is socially expected of them rather than because they are hungry.

The model also identifies three types of activities all of which are closely interrelated to each other and to the 12 activities of living.

Preventing activities These are engaged in to prevent those things which will impair living, such as illness and accidents. Performing acts of personal hygiene to prevent infection, and looking right, left, then right again before crossing the road are examples of preventing activities.

Comforting activities These are performed to give physical, psychological and social comfort. Resting in bed, having hot drinks, and keeping warm when suffering from influenza are examples of comforting activities.

Seeking activities These activities are those carried out in the pursuit of knowledge, new experience and answers to new problems. Going to see the doctor when a symptom is experienced is an example of a seeking activity.

Roper (1976) emphasises the closeness and the overlapping nature of the four types of activities. If a person is suffering illness, he will, by carrying out certain activities of living, seek advice, look for comfort by seeing a doctor and thus try to overcome the illness and prevent it from recurring. All of these concepts combine to form a Model of Living which is illustrated in Figure 5.1.

Activities of living	Lifespan Conception ⟶ Death
Preventing	**Continuum**
Comforting	Totally dependent ⟷ Totally independent
Seeking	
Maintaining a safe environment	_____
Communicating	_____
Breathing	_____
Eating and drinking	_____
Eliminating	_____
Personal cleansing and dressing	_____
Controlling body temperature	_____
Mobilising	_____
Working and playing	_____
Expressing sexuality	_____
Sleeping	_____
Dying	_____

Fig. 5.1 *A model of living (after Roper* et al., *1980).*

The model of living represents the individual — the subject of nursing — engaged in the process of living. Roper (1976) describes the subject of nursing thus:

> Basically, Man is envisaged as carrying out various activities during a life span from conception to death. His main objective is to attain self-fulfillment and maximum independence in each activity of daily living within the limitations set by his particular circumstances. He also carries out many activities of a preventing, comforting and seeking nature and he appropriately alters priorities among the activities of daily living. In these ways, the individual endeavours to be healthy and independent in the process of living.

When the individual is unable to be independent in any of the activities of living, and the family or social grouping is unable to ensure that the activities are performed, nursing is needed.

The goals of nursing

From the model of living developed to describe the individual, it follows that the goals of nursing relate to the activities of living. Nursing aims at:

1. The individual acquiring, maintaining, or restoring maximum independence in the activities of living, or enabling him to cope with dependence on others if circumstances make this necessary.
2. Enabling the individual to carry out preventing activities independently to avoid ill health.
3. Providing comforting strategies to promote recovery and eventual independence.
4. Providing medically prescribed treatments to overcome illness or its symptoms, leading to recovery and eventual independence.

Knowledge and skills for practice

Roper, Logan and Tierney (1980) present a diagrammatic representation of a 'model for nursing' based on the model of living (see Figure 5.2).

Nursing components	Patient's life span
	Conception ⟶ Death
	Totally dependent ⟷ Totally independent
	Circumstance
Activities of living	
Preventing	
Comforting	
Dependent	

Fig. 5.2 *A model of nursing (after Roper* et al., *1980)*

Nurses therefore need knowledge concerning the physiological, sociological and psychological aspects of each of the twelve activities of living, and about the developmental progression along the lifespan; they need the appropriate skills and attitudes to enable them to comfort people, educate them and carry out medical prescriptions to meet 'seeking' and 'preventing' needs; and they need skills to carry out the activities of living for those unable to do so, while helping to cope with dependence in itself.

In order to promote independence in the activities of living, or to actually perform them for others when needed, the model outlines the problem-solving process which nurses follow:

- Assessment of patient
- Identification of patient's problems and statement of expected outcomes

- Planning
- Implementation
- Evaluation

The model therefore suggests that nursing should be based on knowledge of each activity of living, and on the use of the problem-solving process in applying this knowledge to promote independence appropriate to individual circumstances and position on the life span and the dependence/independence continuum.

The essence of the model is presented in Figure 5.3.

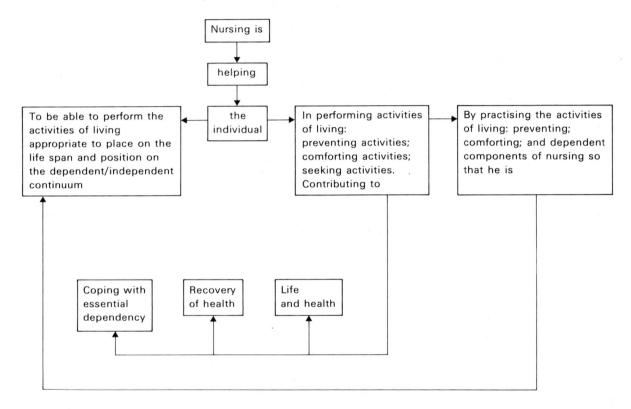

Fig. 5.3 *A diagrammatic representation of the activities of living model.*

Assessment using the activities of living model

Assessment aims at establishing what the patient can and cannot do in each of the activities of living from physical, sociological and psychological perspectives. The 12 activities of living provide the framework for assessment. The patient and nurse discuss each one and identify the usual routine and any obstacles to accomplishment of the usual routine and therefore to independence.

Maintaining a safe environment This refers to seeking and preventing activities, and to the safety of carrying out the activities of living. It may include environmental factors, such as housing and furnishing; sensory factors such as the ability to hear on-coming traffic or to smell gas; personal health-related behaviour such as smoking; and psychosocial factors such as the presence of inappropriate fears or irrational behaviour.

Communicating Through communication itself — between the nurse, the patient and the family — the patient's usual forms of communication and social interaction are established and any difficulties identified. These could include the sensory obstacles of bad hearing or sight.

Breathing Baseline measurements, e.g. respiration count or tidal volume measurement, may be recorded, along with the observation of the colour of mucous membranes and breathing characteristics. Any difficulties related to breathing are identified, as are potentially harmful factors such as smoking.

Eating and drinking This activity embraces cultural attitudes towards food and drink; personal preference; and an assessment of the state of nutrition. Usual eating and drinking patterns are explored, and physical actions such as the ability to cook unaided and to chew food are included.

Eliminating Bowel and bladder functions are discussed under this heading. A record is made of how the patient usually maintains normal function of the bowels and bladder.

Personal cleansing and dressing Again, usual patterns are discussed, such as frequency of baths. Any difficulties in maintaining independence are identified. The condition of the skin, nails and hair would be included in this section.

Controlling body temperature As well as baseline measurement of temperature where appropriate, what the patient usually does to stay warm or become cool would be recorded. For example, if the patient has a coal fire at home, it would be noted, as would the patient's preference for iced drinks when he or she is feeling too hot.

Mobilising The degree of activity and mobility are ascertained, and usual daily activity is recorded. If the patient appears apathetic and reluctant to mobilise, this would be recorded under this heading.

Working and playing The nature of the patient's present or past occupation is recorded, and recreational and relaxational pursuits discussed.

Expressing sexuality Those aspects of sexuality relevant to the current need for nursing are explored. This may include sexual activity in patients with certain medical conditions or disability, and the expression of masculinity and femininity such as dress, make-up etc.

Sleeping The patient's usual sleeping patterns, and the strategies employed by the patient to induce sleep are recorded.

Dying Where appropriate, feelings and views on dying are explored.

Throughout assessment, the activities usually performed independently are recorded, as well as those activities which cannot be performed without assistance. The assessment thus allows the nurse to enable the patient to pursue his or her usual daily life patterns as well as to identify activities which cannot be performed independently. All activities which cannot be independently carried out are treated as problems during assessment. Thus, the organisation of information gathered during assessment using this model is structured around the 12 activities of living described by Roper *et al*. Figure 5.4 is an example of an assessment form developed in a small community unit.

An outline concerning Mr Smith was given on page 52 and we will be returning to him throughout the following chapters. From the perspective of the activities of living model, the assessing nurse noted that Mr Smith 'looked thin' — his clothes were too big for him and he had lost 10 lbs in weight. On asking the patient about his usual activities, it was discovered that he did not eat breakfast and that he had lunch from the Meals-on-wheels service on Tuesdays and Thursdays and from a home help on every other day of the week. He said, however, that he did not eat these lunches and instead had cake and biscuits for tea and only drank cold drinks. He was unable to cook, to make tea safely or to make sandwiches. The assessment therefore showed that the patient was dependent on others for an adequate dietary intake, and that he was unable to cope with this dependence, as suggested by his behaviour in not eating food prepared by others. The other two activities are used to promote exploration to determine an assessment on which to base nursing care.

Care planning

Patient problems relating to the activities of living are identified during assessment and transferred to the plan of care. The goals agreed on by the nurse and patient, when using this model, must relate realistically to those implicit in the model. In other words, the goals must centre around the patient achieving independence in the activities of living *or* coping with any dependencies he or she may have.

The overriding goal is for the patient to agree to the way in which goals are achieved and the schedule for achieving them in as full a way as possible. The model focuses on the behaviour of the individual, and this must be reflected in the problem and goal statements in the care plan. Such an approach is seen as essential to the evaluation of the appropriateness and effectiveness of the nursing

COMMUNITY	
HOSPITAL	
DAY UNIT	

HOSPITAL/UNIT:

PATIENT ASSESSMENT FORM : BASIC DATA

DATE OF ADMISSION	DATE OF ASSESSMENT	NURSE

MALE ☐ AGE ☐

FEMALE ☐ DATE OF BIRTH

SURNAME _____ FORENAMES _____

Prefers to be addressed as

SINGLE/MARRIED/WIDOWED/OTHER

ADDRESS OF USUAL RESIDENCE _____

TYPE OF ACCOMMODATION _____

FAMILY/OTHERS AT THIS RESIDENCE _____

NEXT OF KIN

NAME _____ ADDRESS _____

RELATIONSHIP _____ TEL. NO. _____

SIGNIFICANT OTHERS
(incl. relatives/dependants
visitors/helpers/neighbours) _____

SUPPORT SERVICES _____

OCCUPATION _____

RELIGIOUS BELIEFS & RELEVANT PRACTICES _____

SIGNIFICANT LIFE CRISIS

PATIENT'S PERCEPTION OF CURRENT HEALTH STATUS _____

FAMILY'S PERCEPTION OF PATIENT'S HEALTH STATUS _____

REASON FOR ADMISSION

MEDICAL INFORMATION (e.g. diagnosis, past history, allergies)	WEIGHT _____
	URINE _____
	SG. _____ ALB _____
	TEMP _____ PULSE _____
	B.P. _____ RESP _____
	DISCHARGE ARRANGEMENTS: (to be completed on referral)
MAIN SOURCE FOR ASSESSMENT:	PROJECTED DATE OF DISCHARGE
SIGNIFICANT OTHERS INTERVIEWED : YES/NO	ARRANGEMENTS DISCUSSED WITH:
IF YES, DETAILS OF INTERVIEW	RELATIVES _____ OTHERS _____
	HOME HELP _____
	D/N _____
	H/V _____
	SOC. WORKER

Fig. 5.4 *An assessment form.*

ASSESSMENT OF ACTIVITIES OF LIVING   DATE

AL	USUAL ROUTINES: WHAT HE/SHE CAN AND CANNOT DO INDEPENDENTLY	PATIENT'S PROBLEMS (ACTUAL/POTENTIAL) (P) = POTENTIAL
MAINTAINING A SAFE ENVIRONMENT		
COMMUNICATING		
BREATHING		
EATING AND DRINKING		
ELIMINATING		
PERSONAL CLEANSING AND DRESSING		
CONTROLLING BODY TEMPERATURE		
MOBILISING		
WORKING AND PLAYING		
EXPRESSING SEXUALITY		
SLEEPING		
DYING		

Fig. 5.4 *The assessment form (contd.).*

DATE	ASSESSMENT OUTSTANDING PROBLEMS	DATE	ASSESSMENT OUTSTANDING PROBLEMS

intervention. Figure 5.5 shows how Mr Smith's problems and goals would be recorded following this model.

In this example, nursing has aimed at *preventing* further deterioration in health status, at an adequate intake of food, and at independence in the activity of living concerned — that is eating and drinking. Such independence would, in fact, achieve the other two aims of increasing the daily calorie intake and maintaining weight.

Problem (i.e. lack of independence in activity of living)	Goal (i.e. outcome which will indicate independence or a coping with dependence)
1. Loss of 10 lbs in weight	Weight will remain at same level or rise
2. Intake of less than 1000 calories per day	Will eat at least 1500 calories per day
3. Unable to prepare own meals	Will be able to prepare a meal of his own choice without assistance

Fig. 5.5 *The problem and goal statements.*

The effects of the nursing action taken can be evaluated by comparing the goals with both progress made and the eventual outcome.

The nursing action is what the nurse and patient will do to overcome the problem and achieve the goal. It is a clear description of what the nurse will do to promote independence in the activities of living by carrying out the activities of living, comforting, preventing and dependent components of nursing. (See Figure 5.6.)

Nursing Action
(i.e. how the nurse will promote the patient's independence in the activities of living *or* help the patient to cope with dependence in the process of living)

1. Weigh Mr Smith daily at 9 a.m. He should be wearing his pyjamas.

2. a. Offer choices of food at breakfast, lunch and dinner.

   b. Check how much food is eaten at each meal: estimate calorific value; record; and inform Mr Smith each morning of his estimated calorific intake on the preceding day.

   c. Refer to OT for assessment, provision of aids, and teaching on food preparation.

   d. Ask Mr Smith to make pot of tea at breakfast and tea time in ward kitchen, everyday.

Fig. 5.6 *The nursing action.*

Evaluation focuses on movement towards, or away from the goals of care, and since they are stated in measurable terms the effectiveness of the care can be easily seen.

A patient care study

Mrs Maude Fitzpatrick, an 87 year old woman was referred to the district nursing sister by the general practitioner. On her initial, and the next two subsequent visits, the nurse attempted to assess Mrs Fitzpatrick from the basis of the activities of living model for nursing. In addition to the basic biographical information, the patient's usual patterns of living were assessed with the involvement of her daughter, who was responsible for the performance of some of her mother's activities of living. Problems in the activities of living were identified by the nurse through systematically reviewing all of them. Figure 5.7 shows the written assessment arrived at. The problems identified were used to formulate a plan of care as shown in Figure 5.8.

The focus of the care plan is on the performance of the activities of living — in this case, elimination (problems 1 and 3), personal cleansing and dressing (problem 2), sleeping (problem 3) and communication (problem 4). Those activities of living which were currently being performed independently or being met by the daughter in a way acceptable to her and Mrs Fitzpatrick were not included in the district nurse's plan. It concentrates the patient's energy on the process of living as independently as possible, and on coping with dependence in instances where this is the only realistic alternative. Throughout this account of Mrs Fitzpatrick's care, the emphasis is on the behaviour which people need to engage in to live, within the context of their position on the lifespan, and the dependence/independence continuum. This is the emphasis of the activities of living model, which incorporates the physical, social, and psychological components of behaviour.

	COMMUNITY	✓
	HOSPITAL	
	DAY UNIT	

HOSPITAL/UNIT:

PATIENT ASSESSMENT FORM : BASIC DATA

DATE OF ~~ADMISSION~~ *First visit*	DATE OF ASSESSMENT *2·11·86*	NURSE *Anne Wood*

MALE	☐	AGE *87*	SURNAME *Fitzpatrick*	FORENAMES *Maude Elizabeth*

FEMALE ☒   DATE OF BIRTH *1·8·99*

SINGLE/MARRIED/WIDOWED/OTHER

Prefers to be addressed as *Mrs. Fitzpatrick*

ADDRESS OF USUAL RESIDENCE   *1, The Bungalows, South Milton*

TYPE OF ACCOMMODATION   *2 bedroomed council bungalow. Central heating. No stairs.*

FAMILY/OTHERS AT THIS RESIDENCE   *Daughter*

NEXT OF KIN   NAME *Miss Mary Fitzpatrick*   ADDRESS *as above*

RELATIONSHIP *daughter*   TEL. NO. *None*

SIGNIFICANT OTHERS (incl. relatives/dependants visitors/helpers/neighbours)   *Son – John and family, live in Dorset.*
Mr + Mrs Hardy – next door neighbours.

SUPPORT SERVICES   *Social worker (Nick Hall) Home help (June Timpson) Mon. + Fri.*

OCCUPATION   *Retired from " doing housework for toffs" when 68.*

RELIGIOUS BELIEFS & RELEVANT PRACTICES   *RC priest visits weekly.*

SIGNIFICANT LIFE CRISIS *Loss of husband. "I still mourn for him after 15 years."*

PATIENT'S PERCEPTION OF CURRENT HEALTH STATUS *Has weak bladder + arthritis but "well in herself".*

FAMILY'S PERCEPTION OF PATIENT'S HEALTH STATUS *Daughter says she is worse: senile with poor mobility.*

REASON FOR ~~ADMISSION~~ *Referral*   *Night-time incontinence. Sore under breasts. Help in bath.*

MEDICAL INFORMATION (e.g. diagnosis, past history, allergies)	WEIGHT	*13 stone*	
	URINE	*NAD*	

No apparent medical reason for incontinence – ? due to immobility?

Osteoarthritis of hips and knees for last nine years.

	SG.	ALB
TEMP *37°C*	PULSE *82*	
B.P. *140/90*	RESP *20*	

DISCHARGE ARRANGEMENTS: (to be completed on referral)
Probably needs long-term support.
PROJECTED DATE OF DISCHARGE *Not known.*

MAIN SOURCE FOR ASSESSMENT: *patient and daughter*

SIGNIFICANT OTHERS INTERVIEWED : ⬭YES⬭ NO

ARRANGEMENTS DISCUSSED WITH:

IF YES, DETAILS OF INTERVIEW

Daughter anxious about continuing to care for her mother.

RELATIVES _____   OTHERS _____
HOME HELP _____

D/N _____
H/V _____
SOC. WORKER

Fig. 5.7 *The assessment.*

ASSESSMENT OF ACTIVITIES OF LIVING   DATE 2·11·86

AL	USUAL ROUTINES: WHAT HE/SHE CAN AND CANNOT DO INDEPENDENTLY	PATIENT'S PROBLEMS (ACTUAL/POTENTIAL) (P) = POTENTIAL
MAINTAINING A SAFE ENVIRONMENT	Hangs on To furniture To get around.	
COMMUNICATING	Hears well. Wears glasses.	
BREATHING	Breathes easily and noiselessly.	
EATING AND DRINKING	Wears dentures. Likes toast for breakfast, a cooked lunch, sandwiches for supper. Can't manage tough meat and hard foods. Likes tea and stout.	
ELIMINATING	Opens bowels every other day. Takes Senokot x 2 daily. Dry during the day. Incontinent of urine at night. Can't get up quickly enough at night and usually wets bed x 1.	
PERSONAL CLEANSING AND DRESSING	Can dress herself apart from stockings. Unable To bathe independently - unable To get into bath. Washes own face and hands. Daughter gives wash down weekly.	
CONTROLLING BODY TEMPERATURE	Body temperature normal. House warm - central heating.	
MOBILISING	Walks around house using furniture. Cannot get out alone. Very slow, especially in morning. Difficulty in walking to toilet.	
WORKING AND PLAYING	TV and daily paper. Does no housework.	
EXPRESSING SEXUALITY	Misses husband still.	
SLEEPING	Dozes in afternoon. Bed at 9 p.m. Difficulty in sleeping because of incontinence. Wakes around 2 a.m. and wets bed. Can get back to sleep if daughter changes bed.	
DYING	Wishes she was dead because she is a burden To her daughter, especially since the bed-wetting started.	

Fig. 5.7 The assessment (contd.).

DATE	NO.	PROBLEM	GOAL	NURSING ACTION	REVIEW DATE
2·11·86	1	Incontinence of urine at night because of difficulty in walking.	Will remain dry throughout the night.	1. Change bedtime to 11 p.m. 2. Have her go to toilet before bed. 3. Set alarm for 2 a.m. to wake for toilet. 4. Provide commode at bedside.	9·11·86
	2	Unable to bathe unaided.	Skin will be clean and fresh.	Weekly general bath, using bath seat and step on Thursdays with help of nurse + daughter.	9·11·86
	3	Disturbed sleep because of incontinence.	Will sleep a minimum of 5 hours per night.	Report daily.	9·11·86
	4	Feels she is a burden on her daughter.	Facial expression will be relaxed and she will not mention such feelings in conversation.	Observe and report on moods and conversation.	9·11·86

NAME	NO.	PRIMARY NURSE
Mrs Maude Fitzpatrick	48	Anne Wood

Fig. 5.8 *The care plan.*

6 The Self-care Model for Nursing

The 'self-care' model was developed by Dorothea Orem (Orem 1980), a well-known and respected nurse theorist from the USA. It is a popular model in American nursing, and a number of American nursing schools and their associated units base their curriculum entirely on this model. It is recognised by a growing number of British nurses as a valid description of nursing anywhere.

Based on the issues discussed in Chapters 1–4, the model focuses on the concept of 'self-care'. Although this concept seems, at first sight, to be common sense, it is in fact complex and in many ways very radical. Because of this, it is useful to explore self-care itself, before concentrating on the three parts of the model.

The concept of self-care

Levin *et al.* (1979) define self-care as:

> a process whereby a lay person functions on his/her own behalf in health promotion and prevention, and in disease detection and treatment.

A belief in self-care is therefore associated with a desire to enable and allow people to take the initiative in being responsible for their own health care when this is possible. Although this has, of course, political connotations, there is a desire by ordinary people to be more in control of their lives. Norris (1979) suggests that the idea of self-care first arose in consumer groups in the 1960s, beginning with anti-professional and anti-intellectual feelings, and an urge to return to the kind of life which emphasises 'being human, respecting, and giving'. Norris asks, however, 'But was this really anti-intellectual or simply a reaction to materialism and mechanistic practices?'

Many writers from all spheres, not only health care, support the notion of self-care. In health care, self-care fundamentally affirms that people and families must be allowed to take initiative and responsibility and to develop their own potential in being healthy.

Bennet (1980) says:

> When nurses discuss self care, they need to remember that individuals, healthy and ill, are demanding increased control of their health care. They want to be active in the decision making process: that is, they want to be able to identify their self care needs, to establish their learning goals, and to evaluate their self care behaviour. Patients are rejecting the passive recipient role whereby decisions are made by the nurse, independent of their input. Individuals want to assume responsibility for all aspects of self care.

Self-care is therefore care which is 'given by oneself for oneself'; it is deliberate action, which has an overall purpose related to meeting specific, individual requirements for 'effective living'; it is learned behaviour; and it is aided by intellectual curiosity, instruction and supervision from others, and experience in performing self-care measures. Nurses who accept the concept of self-care as a basis for practice consequently value the patient's right to be regarded as an individual with unique needs, and to be helped to be able to meet their own self-care needs. If one thinks about this carefully, it becomes apparent that promoting self-care is indeed a very radical approach to health care. It means that instead of telling patients what to do, and doing things for them, the nurse actually works towards enabling patients to make decisions and do things for themselves except when this is impossible. Adopting this model is therefore fraught with difficulties, because we, as health workers, have traditionally preferred to place patients in the dependent role:

> The hospital environment itself may be hostile to the goal of reducing patient dependency; nurses dispensing medication by dose, and physicians' refusal to provide medical records to patients are examples. (Norris, 1979)

Predictably, much opposition towards promoting self-care is voiced. One political view sees self-care as a way of pushing responsibility for care back on individuals themselves in an attempt to reduce the need for state provision. Advocates for self-care counter this argument by suggesting that, in fact, the self-care model actually requires as much state resources as the traditional health care system — but it demands that such provisions be used differently. Professionally, handing back enough knowledge to allow informed decision-making by the patient threatens the health care professionals themselves, and Levin *et al.* (1979) say that 'resistance by some health professionals to increased employment of self-care modes is to be expected'.

The customers or potential patients, however, logically argue that when the responsibility for healthy living and health care is vested in the individual and not the professional, the hoped for healthy society is more likely to become part of our reality. There is a rising realisation among American nurses of the enormous potential of developing the self-care concept in nursing. Mullin (1981) describes Orem's self-care nursing model as 'the most liberating and dynamic idea that has been introduced into the practice of medical/surgical nursing for at least twenty years', and says that it 'initiates profound changes in the nurse, the ill adult, and the practice of nursing'.

Understanding Orem's model is easier if these broad issues of self-care are considered before the model itself.

Beliefs and values

The beliefs about humanity in the self-care model of nursing include all those discussed in the introductory chapters, but emphasis is placed on the notion that all individuals have self-care needs, and that they have the right to meet these needs themselves except when this is impossible.

The person who meets the self-care needs is the self-care agent; in the normal, healthy, mature adult this agency is best vested in the individuals themselves. However, the parent is the self-care agent for a newborn infant, and the relative or nurse is the self-care agent for the unconscious person.

Joseph (1980) has presented the six basic premises on which the self-care model for nursing is founded and these in themselves summarise the view of people in relation to self-care:

1. 'Self care is based on voluntary actions which humans are capable of undertaking.

2. Self care is based on deliberate and thoughtful judgement that leads to appropriate acts.

3. Self care is required of every person and is a universal requisite for meeting basic human needs.

4. Adults have the right and responsibility to care for themselves in order to maintain their health, life and well being. Sometimes they may have these responsibilities for others as well, including the children and elderly in a family.

5. Self care is behaviour that evolves through a combination of social and cognitive experience and is learned through one's interpersonal relationships, communications and culture.

6. Self care contributes to the self esteem and self image of a person and is directly affected by self concept.'

Some self-care needs or, in Orem's model, self-care requisites, are universal. That is, they are common to all human beings and are associated with human functioning and life processes. Often referred to as 'basic human needs', the universal self-care requisites are:

- The maintenance of a sufficient intake of air.
- The maintenance of a sufficient intake of water.
- The maintenance of a sufficient intake of food.
- The provision of care associated with elimination processes and excrements.
- The maintenance of a balance between activity and rest.
- The maintenance of a balance between solitude and social interaction.
- The prevention of hazards to human life, human functioning, and human well-being.
- The promotion of human functioning and development within social groups in accordance with human potential, known human limitations, and the human desire to be 'normal'.

Orem describes two further categories of self-care requisites, and these arise out of the influence of events on the universal self-care requisites.

Developmental self-care requisites These occur according to the stage of development of the individual, and the environment in which he or she lives, in terms of its effects on development. They are related to either life changes in the individual or life cycle stages. (See Figure 6.1.)

Health deviation self-care requisites These arise out of ill health and are needs which become apparent because the illness or disability demands a change in self-care behaviour.

When there is a demand to care for oneself, and the individual is able to meet that demand, self-care is possible. But if the demand is greater than the individual's capacity or ability to meet it, an

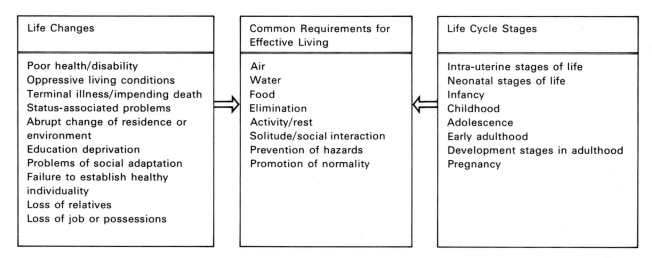

Life Changes	Common Requirements for Effective Living	Life Cycle Stages
Poor health/disability	Air	Intra-uterine stages of life
Oppressive living conditions	Water	Neonatal stages of life
Terminal illness/impending death	Food	Infancy
Status-associated problems	Elimination	Childhood
Abrupt change of residence or	Activity/rest	Adolescence
environment	Solitude/social interaction	Early adulthood
Education deprivation	Prevention of hazards	Development stages in adulthood
Problems of social adaptation	Promotion of normality	Pregnancy
Failure to establish healthy		
individuality		
Loss of relatives		
Loss of job or possessions		

Fig. 6.1 *Developmental influences on self-care in relation to the requirements for effective living (after Pearson and Vaughan, 1984)*

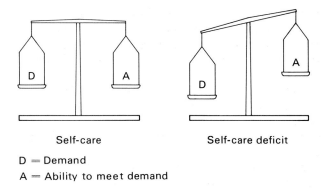

D = Demand
A = Ability to meet demand

Fig. 6.2 *Demand versus ability in self-care.*

imbalance occurs, and this is called a **self-care deficit**. (See Figure 6.2.)

The view of the individual within this model revolves around the fundamental belief that a need for self-care always exists, and that ideally one has the right and ability to meet this need. When the self-care demand is greater than the individual's ability to meet it, the resulting self-care deficit needs to be met. In a newborn baby, the parent acts as the self-care agent, and Orem calls this dependent care. Dependent care is that which is given to someone by a relative, guardian or friend; that is, a meaningful other. If the self-care deficit creates a demand which is more than can be met by self-care and dependent care, nursing in one form or another is required.

The goals of nursing

From this understanding of the person, the goals for nursing logically appear to be the meeting of self-care needs. This can be achieved by:

1. Reducing the self-care demand to a level which the patient is capable of meeting, that is eliminating the self-care deficit.

2. Enabling the patients or clients to increase their ability to meet the self-care demand and thus eliminating any self-care deficits.

3. Enabling the patient or client's meaningful others to give dependent care when self-care is impossible, so that, again, any self-care deficits are eliminated.

4. When none of these can be achieved, by the nurse meeting the individual's self-care needs directly.

Knowledge and skills for practice

Nursing helps people to meet self-care needs by using one of three 'nursing systems', and through five helping methods.

Nursing systems

Totally compensatory nursing system In this system the nurse takes on responsibility for actually carrying out those activities which will meet self-care needs. For example, totally unconscious, acutely ill people will be unable to do many things for themselves, and often relatives are unable to give the needed dependent care.

Partially compensatory nursing system In this system the nurse is still needed to carry out some activities which contribute towards the meeting of self-care needs, but the patient is able to meet some of the needs or a meaningful other can give dependent care. For example, elderly people living at home may be able to meet most of their self-care needs, may receive some dependent care from their family, and may need a nurse to lift them in and out of the bath every week.

Educative/supportive nursing system In this system patients are potentially capable of meeting self-care needs, and the nurse's activity relates to teaching and supporting them so that they will eventually be able to meet the self-care demand. Alternatively, a relative or friend may be helped to give dependent care by the nurse. For example, the newly diagnosed diabetic who needs a daily injection of insulin may well need the nurse to initially give the injection, but the nurse will work towards teaching the patient or a relative how to give the injection.

Nurses help patients using a nursing system, and through five helping methods:

- Acting for or doing for the patient/client.
- Teaching the patient/client.
- Guiding the patient/client.
- Supporting the patient/client.
- Providing an environment in which the patient/client can develop and grow.

To do all this, five main areas for nursing practice are described.

1. Entering into and maintaining nurse patient relationships with individuals, families or groups until patients can be legitimately discharged from nursing.

2. Determining if and how patients can be helped through nursing.

3. Responding to patients' requests, desires and needs for contact with the nurse and assistance.

4. Prescribing, providing and regulating direct help to patients and their family and friends in the form of nursing.

5. Coordinating and integrating nursing with the patient's daily living, other health care needed or being received, and social and educational services needed or being received.

Given the view of the patient/client encompassed in this model, and the way nursing is delivered, it can be seen that a broad knowledge base is required if the goals of the model are to be achieved. The competent nurse needs knowledge about individuals, and each self-care requisite; knowledge and skills related to identifying self-care deficits, prescribing and giving direct care when necessary; and knowledge, skills and attitudes to enable the nurse to work through the five helping methods.

Figure 6.3 is a diagrammatic representation of Orem's self-care model.

Assessment using the self-care model

Assessment from the self-care perspective focuses on the three categories of self-care requisites and aims at identifying self-care deficits. Following assessment, the nurse then proceeds to work together with the patient and the family in planning strategies which will eliminate the deficit by either reducing the self-care demand; increasing the patient's ability to meet the demand; enab-

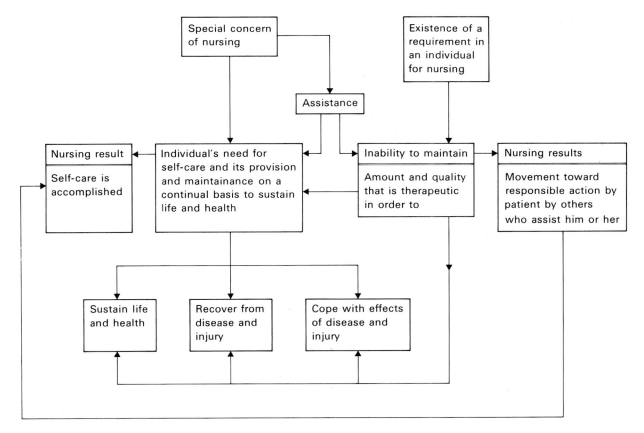

Fig. 6.3 *A diagrammatic representation of Orem's self-care model (after NDCG, 1973).*

NAME: | OTHER PERSONS IMPORTANT TO PATIENT | WHO IS TO BE CONTACTED IN EMERGENCY

ADDRESS:

D.O.B.   M.S.W.   NOK:

Prefers to be addressed as:

Tel:

DOCTOR:

PRIMARY NURSE:

ASSESSMENT – OF SELF-CARE DEFICITS

1. HEALTH DEVIATION SELF CARE REQUISITES

2. UNIVERSAL SELF CARE REQUISITES

MEDICAL INFORMATION

BASE LINE FUNCTIONS

REASON FOR ADMISSION

RELEVANT PAST MEDICAL HISTORY

	Rate	Rhythm	Cough
Breathing			
Circulation			
Pulse Rate	Rhythm	B/P	

Colour   Skin Lips;

MEDICAL DIAGNOSIS

DRUGS TAKEN AT HOME

ALLERGIES

TEMPERATURE   WEIGHT

USUAL PATTERNS CONCERNING DAILY

FLUID INTAKE   cc/mm

ORAL

LIKES

DISLIKES

PATIENT'S FEELINGS & EXPECTATIONS RELATED TO PRESENT ILLNESS

FOOD INTAKE – TYPE, TIME, REGULAR

APPETITE, LIKES DISLIKES

NURSE'S INITIAL IMPRESSION PHYSICAL AND SOCIAL

SPECIAL DIET (WHY?)

IS PATIENT THIN/OBESE/NORMAL

Teeth

Mouth

KNOWLEDGE/INFORMATION/SKILLS NEEDED FOR CONTINUED SELF-CARE AFTER DISCHARGE

PATIENT'S UNDERSTANDING OF ADMISSION

FAMILY'S UNDERSTANDING OF ADMISSION

SOURCE OF ASSESSMENT

SERVICES PROVIDED BEFORE ADMISSION/SERVICES AFTER DISCHARGE

DISTRICT NURSE –

CARE ASSISTANT –

HEALTH VISITOR –

MEALS ON WHEELS –

SOCIAL WORKER –

ANY OTHER –

HOME HELP –

UNIVERSAL SELF-CARE REQUISITES CONT'D

ELIMINATION: CONTINENCE, FREQUENCY, TIMING, COLOUR, AMOUNT, REGULARITY, AIDS NEEDED.

URINE

FAECES

URINALYSIS

CONDITION OF SKIN, NAILS AND HAIR

USUAL PATTERNS OF HYGIENE

SLEEP AND REST, BEDTIME ROUTINE AIDS TO SLEEP

DAILY ACTIVITIES, RECREATION & BODY MOVEMENT

PERSONAL CHARACTERISTICS

BIOLOGICAL RHYTHM BEST TIME/WORST TIME OF DAY

WHAT PATIENT IS ABLE TO DO HIS/HERSELF, WANTS TO DO WITHOUT HELP

WHAT PATIENT WOULD EVENTUALLY LIKE TO DO INDEPENDENTLY

SELF-CONCEPT: BODY IMAGE AND SELF ESTEEM

PAINS OR OTHER SENSATIONS

BALANCE BETWEEN SOLITUDE AND SOCIALISING

COMMUNICATION

FAMILY, FRIENDS, RELATIONSHIPS AND RESPONSIBILITIES

SEXUALITY: INFORMATION ABOUT MARITAL STATUS, RELATIONSHIPS

OCCUPATION AND LIVING ACCOMODATION

DEVELOPMENTAL SELF-CARE REQUISITES: NOTE THE MAJOR LIFE CHANGES, DEVIATION FROM GROWTH AND DEVELOPMENT NORMS: HOW THE PATIENT COPES WITH THEM WHAT OR WHO HELPS HIM/HER (CULTURE, RELIGION, BELIEFS, VALUES)

Fig. 6.4 The assessment form.

ling a meaningful other to give dependent care; or to meet the self-care demand directly.

The aim of assessment is to establish the individual's self-care needs and to identify whether or not there are any self-care deficits. The three groups of self-care requisites can be used as a framework to guide assessment.

Universal self-care requisites

Using observation, measurement and dialogue between the patient and the nurse, normal patterns for the individual related to each of the universal requisites are discovered, and any inabilities to perform self-care are identified and analysed. For example, during assessment of Mr Smith (described on p. 52), the nurse may note signs of weight loss in the patient such as clothes which are too big and loose abdominal skin. The patient himself may tell the nurse that because of the arthritis in his hands he is no longer able to prepare his own food and has to rely on help from the home help and the Meals-on-wheels service for cooked meals. In the past, food preparation has always stimulated his appetite. Weighing the patient shows a loss of 10 lbs.

Thus the assessment shows a self-care deficit in relation to the maintenance of sufficient intake of food which gives rise to the need for nursing action. Currently the home help and Meals-on-wheels service are acting as 'self-care agents' and giving dependent care, but it may be possible for nursing to help the patient to meet his own demand and remove the self-care deficit.

Developmental self-care requisites

In the same way the nurse and patient together identify changes in the patient's life style or life cycle and the developmental needs which arise from these. For example, the growing disability experienced through progressive rheumatoid arthritis leads to a need for acknowledgement on the patient's part that changes in life style are needed. The patient also needs to acquire knowledge and skills to perform self-care acts in a different way and to modify the environment in order to develop new approaches to such acts.

Health deviation self-care requisites

The effects of illness and disease on the individual or observations of behaviour which may lead to illness are considered in this part of the assessment. In this case of a patient who is suffering from rheumatoid arthritis, there may be a range of requisites that need consideration, such as taking appropriate medications, taking a planned diet or supporting affected joints with splints.

The organisation of the recording of the information gathered during assessment can be structured around the three areas of self-care requisites devised by Orem. Figure 6.4 is an example of such a form which was developed by a team of nurses working on a 36-bedded ward and is now currently in use.

Care planning

Once the self-care deficits have been identified from the assessment they can be used as the problem statements on the care plan. The goals established between the nurse and the patient when focusing on self-care must relate realistically to those employed in the model, namely:

- To reduce self-care demand to a level which the patient is capable of meeting.
- To enable the patient to increase his or her ability to meet the self-care demand.
- To enable the patient's relatives or supporters to give dependent care when self-care is impossible.
- To meet the patient's self-care needs directly through nursing when none of the other three alternatives are realistic.

Thus the overriding goal of this model is the elimination of self-care deficits. As in all forms of care planning, both the problem statement and the goal statement should be formulated in such a way as to describe an observable behaviour or measureable entity to allow for evaluation. Figure 6.5 shows how Mr Smith's problem would be recorded using this model.

Problem (i.e. self-care deficit)	Goal (i.e. outcome which will indicate elimination of self-care deficit)
Inability to cook own food because of loss of fine movement in hands	Will be able to prepare a cooked meal of his own choice without help

Fig. 6.5 *The problem and goal statement.*

In this example, nursing has aimed at increasing Mr Smith's own ability to meet the self-care demand. Often, of course, this will not be realistic and other options will have to be selected.

Evaluation of the care can be undertaken by comparing behaviour described in the problem statement with that described in the goal statement. In this case, the patient's initial behaviour was that he could not cook a meal; the goal was that he would be able to perform this action and at evaluation evidence of his ability to do so should be sought.

During the period between the initial assessment and the final assessment of the goal, continuous evaluation revolves around the degree of movement towards or away from the final goal. It may be necessary to modify the nursing action prescribed if movement towards the final goal is not being achieved.

The nursing action is written in a clear and unambiguous way and describes the type of act which the nurse will perform using one or more of the five helping methods:

- Acting for
- Teaching
- Guiding
- Supporting
- Providing a suitable environment

Nursing action (i.e. The act that the nurse will perform to lead to the elimination of the self-care deficit)	Type of Nursing Action

1. Refer to OT for
  a. provision of an apparatus
  b. teaching the use of the aids
	Guiding

2. Discuss possibility of weekly menus and drawing up menu plan	Teaching
3. Weigh weekly on Friday at 9 a.m. in pyjamas	Supporting

Fig. 6.6 *The nursing action.*

Evaluation

If the weight loss continues or if it becomes apparent that there is no progress in his ability to prepare meals, the plan may need to be revised. For example, it could be changed from aiming to enable him to meet his own self-care needs to aiming to assist the home help in acting as the self-care agent, but still including him in the planning and preparing of food. If however, he succeeds in gaining the requisite skills, the self-care deficit will have been eliminated.

A patient care study

Graham Thompson is a 20 year old man admitted to the trauma ward following a road traffic accident where he had sustained a fracture of the left femur. Since he was both physically shocked and in some degree of pain when first admitted, the full assessment was spread over two days using information obtained by both his primary nurse and the associate nurses involved in his care. As in all cases of assessment, the biographical information was recorded as well as the assessment of self-care abilities. Deficits in self-care were recognised by the nurse by systematically assessing all of the self-care requisites identified in the model. Figure 6.7 shows the recordings made during his assessment. From this information the nurse was able to identify Graham's deficits in self-care and thus formulate the care plan.

NAME: *Graham Thompson* D.O.B. *1.12.66* M.S.W. NOK: *Father*

ADDRESS: *12 The Gassens* *Same address*
Highview, Morpeth *and phone*

Prefers to be addressed
as: *Graham*

OTHER PERSONS IMPORTANT TO PATIENT
Girlfriend May Prew

WHO IS TO BE CONTACTED IN EMERGENCY
Father

Tel: *Morpeth 76815*

DOCTOR: *Dr AT Robinson*

ASSESSMENT — OF SELF-CARE DEFICITS

1. HEALTH DEVIATION SELF CARE REQUISITES

2. UNIVERSAL SELF CARE REQUISITES

PRIMARY NURSE:
Paul Peterson

MEDICAL INFORMATION

BASE LINE FUNCTIONS

REASON FOR ADMISSION

*Emergency admission
following crash. Riding
motorbike. Skidded and
hit lamppost. Fractured
left femur and multiple
abrasions to left arm.*

RELEVANT PAST MEDICAL HISTORY

Broken nose 2 years ago

MEDICAL DIAGNOSIS *Fractured left femur*

DRUGS TAKEN AT HOME *None*

ALLERGIES *None*

Breathing	Rate	Rhythm	Cough
	20	*Reg.*	*None*

Circulation *Toes - pink and warm*

Pulse Rate	Rhythm	B/P
76	*Reg.*	*120/70*

Colour Skin Lips:
Nailbeds and extremities - pink.

TEMPERATURE *38°C* WEIGHT *lost 3 lb 3/6*
USUAL PATTERNS CONCERNING DAILY
FLUID INTAKE

ORAL *2500* cc/mm
LIKES *Tea, coffee, lemonade, bitter*
DISLIKES *Milk*
FOOD INTAKE – TYPE, TIME, REGULAR
APPETITE, LIKES DISLIKES
*Cooked breakfast - fried eggs
Lunch - sandwiches
Dinner - meat & vegetables*

SPECIAL DIET (WHY?) *No*
IS PATIENT THIN/OBESE/NORMAL
Teeth *own*
Mouth *clean, moist*

PATIENT'S UNDERSTANDING OF ADMISSION

*"Can't remember much —
I have a broken thigh
bone which will take
about 3 months to knit
together."*

FAMILY'S UNDERSTANDING OF ADMISSION

*"Broken leg, but every-
thing else is alright."*

SOURCE OF ASSESSMENT *Graham*

SERVICES PROVIDED BEFORE
ADMISSION/SERVICES AFTER
DISCHARGE
DISTRICT NURSE –
CARE ASSISTANT –

PATIENT'S FEELINGS & EXPECTATIONS
RELATED TO PRESENT ILLNESS

*Glad he is not worse - expects to
be back to normal in about 4 months.
Expects to get bored.*

NURSE'S INITIAL IMPRESSION
PHYSICAL AND SOCIAL
*Physically "fit"- has lots of friends.
Says "I'll enjoy myself in here, even
if it kills me.*

KNOWLEDGE/INFORMATION/SKILLS NEEDED
FOR CONTINUED SELF-CARE AFTER DISCHARGE

*1. Healing process of bone.
2. Exercises to maintain muscles.
3. Road safety.*

SOCIAL WORKER –
ANY OTHER –

HOME HELP –

HEALTH VISITOR –
MEALS ON WHEELS –

Fig. 6.7 *The assessment.*

UNIVERSAL SELF-CARE REQUISITES CONT'D

ELIMINATION: CONTINENCE, FREQUENCY, TIMING, COLOUR, AMOUNT, REGULARITY, AIDS NEEDED.

URINE
Says it's normal. Dislikes using urinal in bed.

FAECES
Opens bowels, usually daily, in evening.

URINALYSIS
No abnormalities

CONDITION OF SKIN, NAILS AND HAIR
Skin - healthy. Left arm lacerated. Tulle gras and crepe bandage applied in A+E from wrist to shoulder.
Nails - short + clean. Hair on collar. Washes it daily. Dries it with a hair drier.

USUAL PATTERNS OF HYGIENE
Bath - every week day on return from work. Doesn't usually bathe at weekend except if "going somewhere special".

SLEEP AND REST, BEDTIME ROUTINE AIDS TO SLEEP
Goes to bed about midnight. Up at 7am. Mon-Fri, 10-11 a.m. weekends. Goes to sleep "as soon as head touches pillow".

DAILY ACTIVITIES, RECREATION & BODY MOVEMENT
Swims weekly. Football training 2 x week. Pub most nights with mates + girlfriend.

PERSONAL CHARACTERISTICS

BIOLOGICAL RHYTHM BEST TIME/WORST TIME OF DAY
"Hopeless and bad tempered in morning and late at night."

WHAT PATIENT IS ABLE TO DO HIS/HERSELF, WANTS TO DO WITHOUT HELP
Usually independent. While on Thomas Splint he needs all equipment brought to him. Can do everything himself.

WHAT PATIENT WOULD EVENTUALLY LIKE TO DO INDEPENDENTLY
"Everything"

SELF-CONCEPT: BODY IMAGE AND SELF ESTEEM
Appears to have high self esteem and sees himself as "a good looking bloke with a gammy leg."

PAINS OR OTHER SENSATIONS
Cramp in left foot. Otherwise no pain.

BALANCE BETWEEN SOLITUDE AND SOCIALISING
Likes to be with people most of the time. Some privacy when with girlfriend.

COMMUNICATION
Talks easily to people.

FAMILY, FRIENDS, RELATIONSHIPS AND RESPONSIBILITIES
Close to father. Dislikes sister. "Mum is okay." Lives with family.

SEXUALITY: INFORMATION ABOUT MARITAL STATUS, RELATIONSHIPS
Has had same girlfriend for 3 years. She is very important to him. Saving to get married.

OCCUPATION AND LIVING ACCOMODATION
Apprentice plumber- Morpeth District Council. Lives in 3 bedroomed house with upstairs toilet.

DEVELOPMENTAL SELF-CARE REQUISITES: NOTE THE MAJOR LIFE CHANGES, DEVIATION FROM GROWTH AND DEVELOPMENT NORMS: HOW THE PATIENT COPES WITH THEM WHAT OR WHO HELPS HIM/HER (CULTURE, RELIGION, BELIEFS, VALUES)
Wants "own place" as soon as he can marry - and to continue to develop relationship with Mary.

Fig. 6.7 The assessment (contd.).

In this case a deviation in the health care demands, that is the fractured femur he had sustained, led to a deficit in Graham's self-care ability in meeting his universal needs, his development needs and his health deviation needs, as shown on the care plan in Figure 6.8

The focus of the care plan is on teaching Graham to meet as many of his own self-care needs as possible and only acting for him when there is no other alternative. For example, in relationship to his restricted mobility, the nurse's actions concentrate on teaching him the need for movement and methods he can use to help himself, rather than changing Graham's position for him or acting on his behalf.

Health deviation requisites are also recognised. For example, in problems 6 and 7 on the care plan, a lack of knowledge about his own health and the risk of a recurrence of the incident which has led to his admission are identified as problems. In order to help Graham take care of his own health, the nurse's actions emphasise teaching him about his condition and the maintenance of health.

In terms of developmental self-care requisites, the nurse recognises that Graham's injury has interrupted his normal life style and now prevents him from interacting with peers. The reaction he may experience from his friends and the lack of privacy for maintaining important relationships are taken into account in problem 5.

Throughout the descriptions of Graham's care, the issue of encouraging him to function on his own behalf in health promotion, prevention and treatment is highlighted since that is the central focus of the model.

DATE	NO.	PROBLEM	GOAL	NURSING ACTION	REVIEW DATE
	1.	Immobility due to fractured femur + pressure of Thomas splint leading to potential problems of —			
	a.	Breakdown of skin due to pressure + friction.	Intact, unreddened pressure areas.	Explain risks fully. To lift himself off bed using monkey pole for at least 2 min. every hour when awake. Check elbows, heels, sacrum and spinous processes daily at bedmaking. Apply oil to splint ring at 10 a.m. + 6 p.m.	
	b.	Wasting of quadriceps. Thigh girth = 52 cm.	Thigh girth not to fall below 50 cm.	Teach static quadriceps exercises. To exercise and maintain ankle 20 times/hour when awake. Measure thigh at 10 a.m. on Mon. + Thurs.	
NAME			NO.	PRIMARY NURSE	

Fig. 6.8 *The care plan.*

DATE	NO.	PROBLEM	GOAL	NURSING ACTION	REVIEW DATE
	c.	Deep vein thrombosis.	Calf soft and toes pink + warm.	Check calf and circulation to toes at bedmaking time.	
	d.	Constipation.	Daily bowel action.	Vegetables at main meal daily. Record bowel action. If none for 3 days, give aperients as charted.	
	2.	Inability to meet own toilet needs due to immobility.	Can pass urine and faeces when desired.	Leave urinal within easy reach. Give bedpan on request and screen bed. Is able to lift on and off without help. Leave air freshner on locker top.	
	3.	May become bored with restricted activities.	Will say he is reasonably occupied.	Suggest that family provides TV and tape recorder with ear attachment.	
NAME			NO.	PRIMARY NURSE	

Fig. 6.8 The care plan (contd.).

DATE	NO.	PROBLEM	GOAL	NURSING ACTION	REVIEW DATE
	4.	Cramp in left foot.	Any cramp will be relieved in 5 minutes.	Teach ankle exercises to be carried out when cramp occurs. (To circle ankle in full range of movement.) Massage foot when requested.	
	5.	May feel isolated from friends or a lack of privacy.	Will maintain contact with friends. Will have privacy when required.	Encourage friends to visit. Screen bed if desired when girlfriend visits.	
	6.	Lack of knowledge about condition.	Will be able to describe healing process of bone and process of muscle wasting when asked.	Teach, using diagrams - a. structure + healing process of bone. b. structure and function of muscle.	
	7.	Similar injury may occur.	Will not be involved in a similar accident in future.	Teach road safety rules. Give pamphet on road safety to read.	
NAME			NO.	PRIMARY NURSE	

Fig. 6.8 *The care plan (contd.).*

7 | An Adaptation Model for Nursing

The model for nursing described by Sister Callista Roy was developed throughout the 1960s and first put into use in a degree nursing programme in California in 1970. It is now quite widely used in that state and it has also been adopted for use in a few clinical units in the United Kingdom.

The model is largely based on systems theory although it does take into account some thoughts from interactionist theory. The framework from which it has been developed is the way in which an individual, as a whole system, responds or *adapts* to changes or *stimuli*, whether the stimuli are within the individual or in the surrounding environment.

The theory on which Roy has based this model of nursing is complex but well supported by scientific evidence. Its underlying framework is easily identified. She clearly states the assumptions or beliefs on which the model is based, the goals she sees nurses as trying to achieve, and the knowledge they require in order to do so. In describing how the model may be put into use, she uses a problem-solving approach recommending a clear guide for assessment, problem identification, the setting of goals, and the planning, implementation and evaluation of care. She also gives some guidance on the setting of priorities. Her rationale for using this model is that it not only enhances a client-centred approach but also allows for the professional accountability of nursing as a scientific, service-oriented discipline.

Beliefs and values

Roy (1976) herself points out that the beliefs on which this model is based may not be scientifically proved but have been accepted as being true. They concern the view of people as individuals and the way they interact with the environment. Rambo (1984) clearly describes these assumptions, an understanding of which is the key to the remainder of the model. These assumptions include the following:

1. Each person is seen as an integrated whole, with biological,

psychological and social components, and in constant interaction with the surrounding environment.

2. In order to maintain homeostasis or integrity, people must respond or adapt to any changes that occur using both innate and acquired mechanisms.

3. The changes or stimuli which affect people can be divided into three types:

Focal — those things which immediately affect them such as a chest infection, a bereavement or a new baby.

Contextual — all the other stimuli present at the time which may influence a negative response to the focal stimulus, such as anaemia, poor housing or social isolation. They are the surrounding circumstances.

Residual stimuli — these are the beliefs, attitudes and traits of an individual, developed from the past but affecting the current response. For instance, one person's upbringing may teach him or her to tolerate low back pain without complaint, while another person might consider it abnormal and require treatment for it.

4. Every person has what is known as an individual adaptation zone which is concerned with his or her capacity to respond to stimuli. Provided that all the stimuli that affect individuals fall within that zone, the responses they make to them will maintain their integrity and are seen as adaptive or positive. If however the stimuli are too great, the adaptations made in response will not be able to maintain integrity and are seen as maladaptive or negative.

The size of an individual's adaptive zone is personal and varies from person to person. For instance, under the pressure of pending examinations, one individual may adapt by following a pre-planned revision schedule, a positive adaptation within the personal zone. Another may respond by sleeplessness, poor concentration and loss of appetite, a negative adaptation outside his personal zone.

5. All people have certain needs which they endeavour to meet in order to maintain integrity. Roy divides these needs into four different modes:

Physiological — associated with the structure of the body and the way it functions.

Self-concept — concerned with the way one perceives oneself, with mental activity and with the expression of feelings.

Role function — concerned with the psychosocial wholeness in fulfilling one's own role and society's expectations of various roles.

Interdependence — the balance between dependence on others and independence in achieving things for oneself.

6. An individual's ability to remain healthy is dependent on having sufficient energy and ability to make positive adaptations to stimuli. Illness occurs when the responses made fall outside an individual's adaptation zone either because there is insufficient energy or the stimulus is too great. Health and illness are seen as lying on a continuum, and movement along this continuum is an inevitable part of life.

Some of the terms which Roy uses to describe the assumptions or beliefs of this model may not be familiar and often require two or three readings before they can be used with ease. Nevertheless they are worth pursuing since once mastered, they provide a very useful basis on which to build a model for practice.

The goals of nursing

In Roy's view the purpose of nursing is to help people to adapt to stimuli in any of the four categories identified in order to help them free energy to respond to other stimuli. She suggests that a goal statement should include the behaviour which is to be changed and the direction of the change. She also emphasises that since it is the behaviour of the patient or client which is to be changed, he or she must be involved in identifying goals whenever possible.

If Roy's assumptions are to be believed, then human behaviour is constantly directed towards an attempt to maintain integrity or homeostasis. In many instances, whether or not this has been achieved can be judged by a knowledge of *norms*. Such knowledge can also be used to help patients to identify their own goals.

It must, however, be pointed out that *norms* are only guidelines and may vary among individuals or in different societies. For instance while some physiological norms are fairly constant for all people, such as the levels of potassium in the blood, others may vary widely such as the frequency of elimination. Similarly, what is a socially acceptable way of behaving in one society may be unacceptable in another.

To summarise the goals of nursing according to Roy's model, they are:

- Related to achieving adaptive responses in the physiological, self-concept, role function and interdependence modes.
- Stated in behavioural terms.
- Guided by a knowledge of 'norms'.
- Planned in conjunction with the patient.

Knowledge and skills for practice

The knowledge base on which Roy's model is built obviously relates to her views about people and the goals of nursing. It can be divided into four main sections, associated with the four adaptive modes, namely the physiological, self-concept, role function and inter-dependence modes, each of which will be briefly outlined here.

Physical mode

Roy identifies six basic physiological needs that have to be met in order to maintain integrity. They are:

- Exercise and rest
- Nutrition
- Elimination
- Fluid and electrolytes
- Oxygenation and circulation
- Regulation of temperature, senses and the endocrine system

In each area it is necessary to have knowledge of body structure and function, the standards or ranges which are accepted as normal, the stresses which can affect them, and the sort of maladaptive behaviour which may occur.

Self-concept

As Rambo (1984) points out, self-concept is a difficult thing to explain, but when related to adaptation nursing it 'consists of feelings and beliefs that permit an individual to know who he or she is and feel that the self is adequate in meeting needs and desires'.

Broadly, self-concept is divided into two parts. The physical self is concerned with how people actually perceive themselves in relationship to their feelings, sensations, appearance and body image. Difficulties in this area are often experienced as a feeling of loss, such as might occur following mutilating surgery, or even the perceived loss of sexual ability following myocardial infarction. The personal self is concerned with consistency of personal standards and behaviours, ideals and moral ethical issues. Feelings of anxiety, powerlessness or guilt may alert you to difficulties in this area.

Role function

Roy (1976) describes role as 'the title given to the individual — mother, son, student, carpenter — as well as the behaviours that society expects an individual to perform in order to maintain the title'.

The idea of a 'role tree' has been used by Rambo (1984) to clarify the subject. (See Figure 7.1.) The trunk of the tree represents the

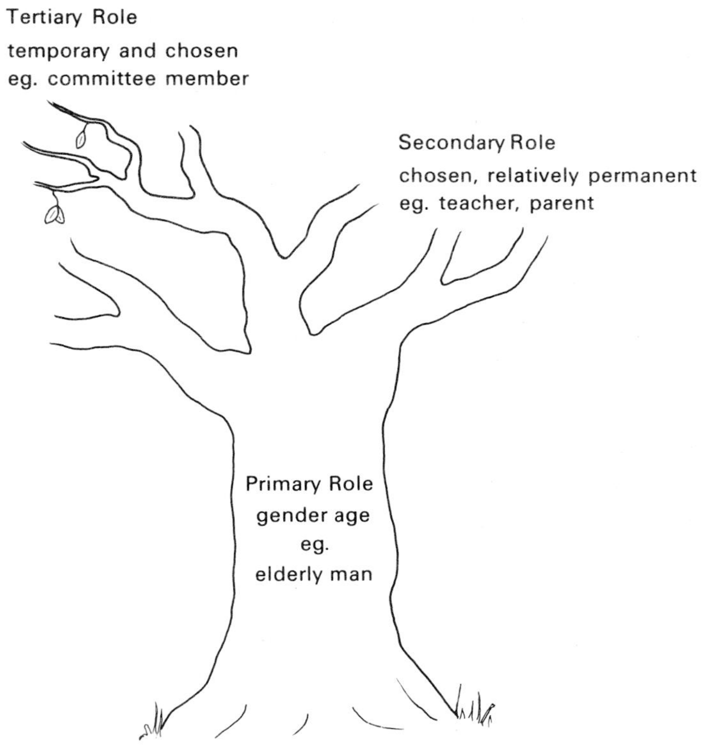

Tertiary Role
temporary and chosen
eg. committee member

Secondary Role
chosen, relatively permanent
eg. teacher, parent

Primary Role
gender age
eg.
elderly man

Fig. 7.1 *The role tree.*

primary, relatively consistent pre-determined role of an individual; it is related to gender and age group such as adolescent girl or elderly man. The branches represent the secondary roles which are relatively permanent, may be chosen, and are linked with stages of life such as parent, engineer, student or spouse. The leaves of the tree represent tertiary roles which are usually temporary, freely chosen and relatively minor. Examples may include committee member, tennis player or club secretary.

It is often sudden change in secondary roles which may lead to difficulties such as may occur with a new job, a sudden bereavement or parenthood. Inability to master a role; conflict between two roles; or too many roles are all things to be on the alert for as potentially problematic.

Interdependence

The final area of knowledge which is related to this model pertains to the mode of interdependence, the fine balance between dependence on others and independence. Dependence is demonstrated by a need for affiliation with others, for their care, support and approval. Independence is demonstrated by the ability to achieve, make decisions and initiate actions by oneself. Interdependence is seen as a balance between the two extremes of taking and giving, the ability to stand alone but not be so fiercely independent that sharing with others becomes impossible. Figure 7.2 is a diagrammatic representation of Roy's adaptation model for nursing.

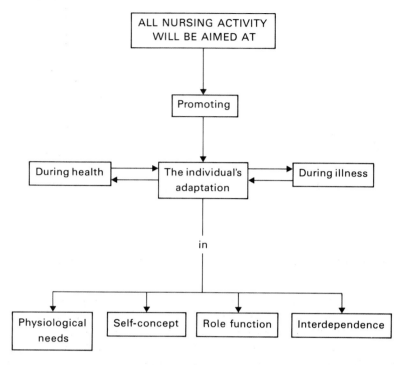

Fig. 7.2 *A diagrammatic representation of Roy's adaptation model (after NDCG, 1973).*

Assessment using an adaptation model

The focus of this model is adaptation and the aim of assessment is two-fold: to identify the actual and potential behaviours of the client which are seen as maladaptive or inappropriate, and to identify the stimuli or causes of the maladaptive behaviour.

The four adaptation modes can be used as the basic framework to guide assessment. These modes again are the physiological, self-concept, role function and interdependence modes.

Roy recommends that assessment has two distinct parts. First level assessment is concerned with describing the current behaviour of the patient, while second level assessment is concerned with the factors, the stimuli, which have caused that behaviour.

First level assessment

This is the stage of the nursing process at which data is collected and a judgement is made as to whether it is adaptive or maladaptive. Within each of the four modes are basic human needs which can be

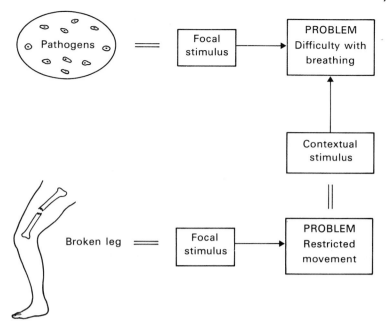

Fig. 7.3 *A single stressor identified as both a focal and contextual stimulus.*

affected by either deficits or excesses, for example, too little oxygen, too high a blood sugar or too much dependency. The nurse uses interview, observation and measurement skills to assess the current behaviour of the patient in each of the four modes and, based on this assessment, makes a tentative judgement as to whether the behaviour is adaptive, maladaptive or potentially maladaptive.

Second level assessment

This is the stage of assessment at which the cause of the behaviour is identified. It is an essential step since the nursing actions are based on the information gained. The stimuli affecting the patient's behaviour are identified in the three groups discussed earlier in this chapter, namely focal stimuli, contextual or surrounding stimuli, and residual stimuli. In some instances the focal stimulus of one patient's problem may be the contextual stimulus of another and this may initially lead to some confusion. For example, the focal stimulus of a problem of difficulty with breathing may be the presence of a chest infection and the contextual stimulus may be a broken leg causing restricted movement. However, the broken leg itself will be the focal stimulus or a direct cause of the behavioural problem of immobility. (See Figure 7.3.) However, as with any other assessment guide, the user soon overcomes this difficulty and develops a clear pattern for use.

Information may be gathered from the patient him or herself, from friends or relatives, from other health care workers or from laboratory findings.

Considering Mr Smith's assessment and his problem of weight loss, information can be gathered about each of the four adaptive modes, using the adaptation framework.

Physiological

At first level assessment, the nurse may observe that Mr Smith appears thin and has loose fitting clothes. During the interview she may ascertain that his nutritional intake is low, that he has no appetite and that his weight has fallen by 10 lbs. This will lead to the recognition that he has a behavioural problem which is maladaptive in relationship to his nutritional needs. Proceeding to second level assessment, the nurse will attempt to ascertain why the weight loss has occurred since this will give her information about the focus of her nursing intervention. At this stage she may discover his inability to prepare his own food due to the limitations arising from his rheumatoid arthritis. This information is recorded as shown in Figure 7.4.

Patient Behaviour	Stimulus		
	Focal	Contextual	Residual
Loss of 10 lb in weight over last 3 months	Inability to prepare own food	Loss of fine hand movement due to rheumatoid arthritis	

Fig. 7.4 *A care plan item — physiological.*

Self-concept

During conversation the nurse may ascertain that Mr Smith has always enjoyed preparing his own meals and that his inability to do so at the moment has left a gap in his life. He describes feelings of loss about his ability to be able to cook for himself which to him has always been important for developing an appetite for food. Using this information the nurse may perceive a problem related to self-concept, a feeling of loss of ability. (See Figure 7.5.)

Patient Behaviour	Stimulus		
	Focal	Contextual	Residual
Upset at not being able to cook own food	Loss of ability to cook	Cooking is an integral part of his normal lifestyle	

Fig. 7.5 *A care plan item — self-concept.*

Role function

A secondary role function for Mr Smith has been that of cooking his own food, which is currently lost. The nurse observes that he has not been able to adjust to changes in his ability to maintain this role through alterations caused by his rheumatoid arthritis. (See Figure 7.6.)

Patient Behaviour	Stimulus		
	Focal	Contextual	Residual
Does not eat food prepared by other people	Has always seen himself as the 'best cook'	Dislikes accepting support from others	Has lived alone for 20 years

Fig. 7.6 *A care plan item — role function.*

Interdependence

The focus of assessment in this area is the balance between giving and taking actions. Through discussion with Mr Smith, the nurse may perceive that all his life he has been independent of others and unwilling to accept help. The dependence caused by his reliance on others for help in preparing food has led to difficulty in his accepting any help. (See Figure 7.7.)

Patient Behaviour	Stimulus		
	Focal	Contextual	Residual
Mr Smith says he dislikes accepting any help from the 'welfare'	Has always lived independently and dislikes help from others	No longer able to meet nutritional needs independently	

Fig. 7.7 *A care plan item — interdependence.*

It is fairly easy to structure a formal assessment form using the framework that Roy suggests. Following a section for biographical and medical information, the four adaptation modes that she has identified can be used as main headings with sub-sections of the components of each one. However, provided that the nurse is familiar with the content of the model, an alternative would be to use a freer format. In this way the emphasis of the assessment can be directed towards the major areas of concern of the patient without becoming too bulky or wasting space. Figure 7.8 is an example of an assessment form which follows a more formal structure, demonstrating how information relating to both individual strengths and areas giving rise to difficulties can be gathered. In this way the areas of strength can be drawn upon when formulating a plan of action. Information concerning biographical data follows a simple standard format. (See Figure 7.8.)

Ward	Admission Date	House Officer	Consultant
		Reason for Admission	G.P.	Tel. No.'s
			Social Worker
		Surgery / Treatment	Relatives Staying
Age	Marital Status		
D.O.B.	Occupation		
Religion	Baptised	Patient's Understanding of Admission	Dependants/Siblings
Likes to be Referred to as			

NEXT OF KIN	Tel. No.'s		DISCHARGE ARRANGEMENTS	
Name		Family's Understanding of Admission	Needed	Ordered
Address			Out-Patients	
			District Nurse	
			Convalescence	
Meaningful Others		Relevant Past Medical History	Health Visitor	
			Home Help	
			Transport	
			Discharge Advice	
TYPE OF ADMISSION			TTO's	
Emergency / Waiting List			Others	
Provisional Medical Diagnosis				
		Allergies/Infectious Diseases	Drugs Taken At Home	
Actual Medical Diagnosis				
			Discharge Date	

Fig. 7.8 The assessment form.

Modes	Behaviour	Stimuli		
		Focal	Contextual	Residual
PHYSIOLOGICAL 1. Oxygen & Circulation:				
2. Fluid & Electrolytes:				
3. Elimination:				
4. Nutrition:				
5. Rest/Activity:				
6. Regulation:				

Fig. 7.8 *The assessment form (contd.).*

Modes	Behaviour	Stimuli		
		Focal	Contextural	Residual
SELF-CONCEPT 1. Physical self:				
2. Personal self:				
ROLE FUNCTION 1. Primary:				
2. Secondary				
3. Tertiary				
INTERDEPENDENCE 1.				
2.				

The amount of space in each section can be adjusted according to the
particular needs of each unit.

Fig. 7.8 *The assessment form (contd.).*

Care planning

Although both adaptive and maladaptive behaviour may be recorded during assessment, the identification of problems arises out of the actual or potential maladaptive behaviour. The goals focus on an adjustment of the maladaptive behaviour to lie within the norms, whether those norms are universal as in such things as temperature, or individual as may be the case in eating habits. Since the goal of nursing is aimed towards adjusting the patient's behaviour to be within these norms, great emphasis is placed on formulating them jointly with the patient. Thus the overriding goal in this model is that the patient should move towards adaptive behaviour. Because of the recognition of a need to evaluate the effectiveness of care, the problems and goals are always stated in behavioural terms which can either be observed or measured. (See Figure 7.9.)

Problem (i.e. maladaptive behaviour)	Goal (i.e. adaptive behaviour)
Weight loss caused by a. inability to cook own food b. loss of appetite	Able to eat sufficient food to maintain weight

Fig. 7.9 *Planning care.*

In this example the goal is related to producing a demonstration of positive or adaptive behaviour. Evaluation will be undertaken by measuring the weight at predetermined intervals to ascertain whether it has become stable and by recording the amount of food eaten.

The nursing action is aimed towards adjusting the stimuli which have led to the maladaptive behaviour. This is why it is so essential to identify these causes during second level assessment. If the stimulus is unalterable, it may be necessary for the nurse to intervene on behalf of the patient. (See Figure 7.10.)

Nursing Action (ie. alteration of the stimuli which have led to the maladaptive behaviour)

1. Refer to occupational therapist for
 	
   a. provision of appropriate aids
   b. teaching use of aids
 	
2. Discuss possible weekly menus and draft a sample with Mr Smith
 	
3. Weigh weekly on Fridays at 9.00 a.m. in pyjamas

Fig. 7.10 *The nursing action.*

Further problems would be identified from the information gathered at assessment in relationship to Mr Smith's loss of independence, self-concept and role function and dealt with in a similar way.

A patient care study

Tracey Foster is a 21 year old girl admitted from the waiting list to a busy acute general surgical ward. She has been attended by her general practitioner for episodes of biliary colic and has undergone a cholecystogram which has confirmed the presence of gall stones.

Tracey's assessment was undertaken on the morning of admission. The amount of recording is relatively short as it is recognised that in this type of situation time is limited. However, even in this situation, it is possible to record all information essential to care in a relatively brief way.

The biographical data is recorded on a format which can be used fairly universally. However, the data related to adaptive and maladaptive behaviour is recorded using the format suggested by Roy of both first and second level assessment and recording both the behaviour and the cause of the behaviour. Figure 7.11 shows the recordings made during Tracey's assessment.

From the data collected the nurse was able to identify both actual and potential maladaptive behaviour or problems and continue to formulate the care plan. In this case maladaptive behaviour in all four modes was identified, although some of the problems overlapped as shown in the care plan in Figure 7.12. The nursing action is planned in accordance with the stimuli which have been identified as leading to the problems. For instance, problem 1 relates to the risk of chest infection, a physiological difficulty caused by smoking habits and impending anaesthesia. The action is aimed towards altering the smoking habits and providing preventative support to lessen the risks during anaesthesia.

Problem 4 relates to difficulties which were ascertained through assessment of the role function and interdependence modes and action is again planned around the identified courses.

The whole emphasis of this study has been on the identification of adaptive and maladaptive behaviour; on the stimuli leading to this behaviour and the way in which the nurse can help the patient to manage the stimuli in order to attain positive adaptation. The overall goal can be seen as maintaining integrity or homeostasis and the actions are focused around manipulating the stimuli in such a way as to achieve this goal. The resultant plan is easy to follow, with very clear guidance on the type of behaviour to be looked for during evaluation, thus enabling the nurse to make a judgement about both the accuracy of her assessment and the effectiveness of her planned intervention.

Ward Roy	Admission Date 12.7.84	House Officer Dr Arnold	Consultant Dr Deacon
Tracey Foster Flat 12 Hamlet House 22 South Street Acton		Reason for Admission *Episodes of biliary colic caused by gall stones.*	G.P. Dr Smith Tel. No's 82715
		Surgery / Treatment *For cholecystectomy 13.7.84*	Social Worker None
Age 21 Marital Status Single			Relatives Staying No
D.O.B. 23.4.63 Occupation Typist		Patient's Understanding of Admission	
Religion C of E Baptised		"My gall bladder is blocked with stones which keep giving me awful pains. I need them out."	Dependants/Siblings None
Likes to be Referred to as Tracey			
NEXT OF KIN Parents Tel. No's None		Family's Understanding of Admission	DISCHARGE ARRANGEMENTS

			Needed	Ordered
Name Mr & Mrs Foster		As above.	Out-Patients	
Address 31 The High Street Acton			District Nurse	
			Convalescence	
Meaningful Others		Relevant Past Medical History	Health Visitor	
Barbara Smith, Sue Kelland (Flatmates)		Nil relevant.	Home Help	
Flat 2, Hamlet Hse, 22 South St. Tel 78326		No previous hospital admission.	Transport	
TYPE OF ADMISSION			Discharge Advice	
Emergency / Waiting List Waiting list			TTO's	
Provisional Medical Diagnosis			Others	

	Allergies/Infectious Diseases	Drugs Taken At Home	
Actual Medical Diagnosis	None.	Paracetamol occasionally for headaches and pains. Had pethidine for biliary colic with effect	
Intermittent biliary colic from gall stones. Confirmed by cholecystogram.			Discharge Date

Fig. 7.11 The assessment form.

Modes	Behaviour	Stimuli		
		Focal	Contextual	Residual
PHYSIOLOGICAL 1. Oxygen & Circulation:	No current difficulty but smokes 10 cigarettes a day.	Cigarette smoke is an irritant to breathing.	For anaesthetic tomorrow. Breathing may be restricted by pain postoperatively.	Family all smoke.
2. Fluid & Electrolytes:	No observed difficulties.			
3. Elimination:	Opens bowels daily after breakfast. No difficulty with micturition. Urine testing-NAD.			
4. Nutrition:	Conscious of figure but enjoys food. Eats balanced diet. Pain and nausea if fatty foods eaten.	Bile flow to gut impaired. Limited knowledge of cause of pain.		
5. Rest/Activity:	Usually sleeps well but currently cannot get off to sleep.	Anxious about impending surgery.	Unfamiliar surroundings.	
6. Regulation:	No difficulties noted: T 36.8°C BP 120/70 P 72			

Fig. 7.11 *The assessment form (contd.).*

Modes	Behaviour	Stimuli		
		Focal	Contextural	Residual
SELF-CONCEPT 1. Physical self:	Says she is concerned about appearance of scar.	Impending surgery will leave scar.	No previous surgical scars.	Mother has large scar from surgery 20 years ago.
2. Personal self:	Concerned that she "won't be brave".	No previous experience of surgery.	Cries easily.	
ROLE FUNCTION 1. Primary:	Young woman.			
2. Secondary	New job as a typist. Anxious about not being able to work for 4-6 weeks.	Requires sick leave following surgery.	Feels insecure in new job.	Father is unemployed at present.
3. Tertiary	Swims weekly. Likes pop music and discos.			
INTERDEPENDENCE 1.	Freedom restricted by hospitalisation.	Never been in hospital before.		Dislikes new surroundings.
2.	Plans to convalesce with family.	Has been living with 2 friends in flat for 6 months.	Family unhappy about moving out of home.	Sister did not move from home until married.

The amount of space in each section can be adjusted according to the particular needs of each unit.

Fig. 7.11 *The assessment form (contd.).*

	NURSING RECORD		
CARE PLAN_____		MR/MRS(MISS) *Tracey Foster*	

Admissions Care Plan

Date	Problems — Actual (A) and Potential (P)	Desired Outcome	Nursing Action
12·7·84	1. (P) Chest infection due to smoking habit and impending surgery.	Respiratory rate not more than 18/min. No cough.	Refer to physiotherapist for deep breathing exercises. Supervise breathing exercises hourly when awake. Advise to restrict or, if possible, stop smoking.
	2. (P) Pain and nausea if fatty foods are eaten.	Will not complain of pain or nausea.	Fat free diet prior to surgery.
	3. (A) Unable to sleep due to anxiety and strange environment.	Will sleep minimum of 6 undisturbed hours at night.	Warm milk at bed time. Offer sedatives as charted if desired.
	Anxiety due to: a) surgical scar. b) ability to cope. c) security of job. d) temporary loss of independence.	Is able to discuss anxieties freely in a relaxed way.	a) Describe likely progress of surgical scar. Show photos of previous patients' scars. b) Discuss fears about surgery and explain postoperative management of pain etc. Offer her time to ask questions.

Fig. 7.12 *The care plan.*

8 The Health Care Systems Model for Nursing

The origins of this model lie in a concern for the need to develop a broad-based conceptual framework for curriculum design, which would provide unity, coordination and integration of the nursing course content (Neuman, Young, 1972). The author of the model, American nursing theorist Betty Neuman, has moved away from the traditional 'illness' model to one which encompasses a 'total person approach to patient care'. The strength of her model lies in the emphasis given to prevention, health education and wellness as well as to the management of ill health and the interdisciplinary approach.

Neuman (1980) suggests that this model is not restricted to nursing but can be shared by anyone working in health care systems. Indeed this is one of its great strengths in that, rather than fragmenting care, it offers an interdisciplinary approach and pulls together the goals and emphases of many disciplines concerned with health care. It stresses the complementary work of doctors and nurses within society and suggests that nurses should broaden rather than restrict their input. While Neuman is quite clear in seeing a unique role for nursing, Craddock and Stanhope (1980) suggest that her model is not clear in pointing out what that role is. However, they find the model helpful in identifying clients' needs for health care and suggest that in using this approach, the nursing role has potential for developing more independently. But, they continue to warn: 'If in fact this does not occur the nurse must become an endangered species . . . in the present health care system the nurse's functions have been parcelled out to other professionals . . . the nurse's distinct contribution is obliterated'.

Neuman and Wyatt (1981) also express some concern about the nursing role, recognising the danger of a split between what they call the 'technical' and the 'professional' nurse. They see the role of the nurse as the caring, collaborating and coordinating health care worker and feel that the model that is described here supports these functions.

Neuman has drawn on several theories in developing the health care systems model. Systems theory and stress adaptation have been described earlier. There is also evidence of Gestalt and field theories.

These emphasise how we normally live in a carefully balanced equilibrium. If a problem arises, tension occurs and disrupts the equilibrium. This disruption is the driving force which leads us to interact with our environment and adapt or change. Components of developmental theory can also be recognised. Although originally devised for use in curriculum development, the model has been tried and tested in clinical settings and as a framework for management. While the evaluation of its use in these settings has highlighted some minor difficulties, it seems to have been found helpful in both areas.

Beliefs and values

There is a very strong emphasis in this model on viewing the individual as a whole person who is affected by all the variables that can impinge on human beings. People are seen as open systems in constant interaction with their environment.

Neuman (1980) recognises that there are common features in any species and that there is a core of such features in people. This central core or central structure is a person's energy resource and if it is compromised that person is at risk. The core is made up of basic survival factors, such as physiological, anatomical and genetic features. There is however a range of unique variables within this common core giving each person his or her own individual baseline. For example, while all human beings require sufficient pressure to circulate the blood, the actual degree of pressure may vary considerably from person to person.

Surrounding this basic energy resource are lines of resistance which protect it in order that it can remain stable. The lines of resistance may be such things as immune defences, coping behaviours or physiological mechanisms. They can vary from person to person according to the stage of development, the life style or past experience. Their function is to help individuals maintain a harmony between the internal and external factors in their environment. In total they form an individual's normal line of defence which is a relatively stable state which has been developed over a period of time. This line is partly acquired through the responses or adaptations which have been experienced previously. For example, someone who has suffered from measles in the past will have acquired immunity against the virus and be able to resist future exposures. Similarly, past experience of successfully preparing for examinations will lead to the ability to cope with future exposures to this situation.

Surrounding this normal line of defence is also a flexible line of defence which Neuman likens to an accordian. It can vary from day to day and can be affected by such things as the amount of rest, the nutritional state, or the number of interactions that are occurring at that particular point in time. For example, a mother who is tired following a birth of a second child may be less tolerant of the attention sought by her first child. Similarly there is a known

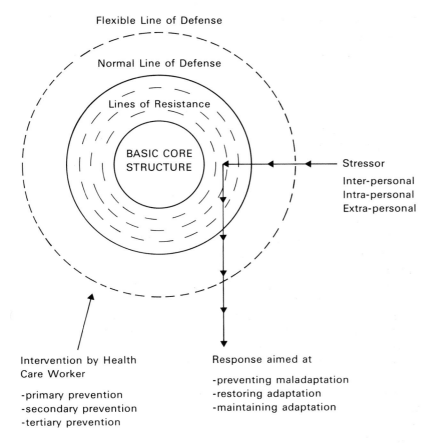

Fig. 8.1 *The health care systems model (simplified).*

association between stressful life events such as a divorce or a change of job and physical illness. At a simpler level, a late night may well lead to less tolerant behaviour the following day. The variables which can affect these lines of defence arise from physiological, psychological, sociocultural and developmental sources.

Throughout a life span each person is subject to stressors which are seen as stimuli which produce tension within the system. The tension has potential to cause a disequilibrium or a disturbance in the harmony of the individual and they require a response. The lines of defence respond to the stressors to prevent them from reaching the central energy resource since, if this is impinged upon, life is threatened. Stressors can be divided into three categories:

Intrapersonal These occur within the individual. As well as stressors related to disease, infection or trauma, conditioned responses to life events such as grief, or developmental changes are included in this category.

Interpersonal These occur between one or more other people. Events such as conflict within a family, role changes and dependency may be included here.

Extrapersonal These occur outside the individual. Circumstances of poverty, deprivation, educational systems or cultural changes are classified as extrapersonal stressors.

Many stressors are universal and will always affect people. An example of such a stressor is loss which can affect us all even if we have developed different lines of defence and respond differently. Other stressors, however, will only have meaning to the individual concerned, and so they have to be viewed from his or her own perception of them rather than the health care worker's perception. This is of vital importance in understanding how to apply the model in practice. The response to a stressor varies from individual to individual according to how effective the lines of defence are in that particular situation, and how much disruption occurs within the system. The responses to stressors can also occur at intrapersonal, interpersonal or extrapersonal levels. For example, a family quarrel can lead to intrapersonal changes such as loss of sleep, interpersonal changes such as poor family communications, and extrapersonal changes such as loss of earnings from difficulty in concentrating at work.

The goals of nursing

The broad goal that is sought in this model is the stability of the system — that is, the whole person. Again there are three categories that goals can be placed in. These link with the situation and the foci of the intervention. They are related to preventing maladaptation, restoring adaptation and maintaining adaptation.

Primary prevention If a stressor is suspected or identified before a reaction with the system occurs, the goal of care is to either reduce the possibility of an encounter with the stressor or to strengthen the line of defence in order that a reaction can be reduced or stopped. This area of care links strongly with current trends in both preventative care and health education. It would include such things as immunisation programmes and education about relaxation techniques and managing one's own health. Its prime purpose is to prevent maladaptation occurring.

Secondary prevention This type of intervention occurs after a stressor has crossed the line of defence and caused a reaction. In this instance the goal of care is aimed towards helping an individual to return to his own normal health state or, to use Neuman's terms, to reconstitute. She emphasises that what is seen as healthy for one person may not be the same as for another. At this stage the focus of intervention is to restore adaptation and stability.

Tertiary prevention The third type of intervention is generally started after the 'treatment stage'. Its purpose is in helping a person to maintain or stabilise his or her healthy state in order to avoid the possibility of a recurrance of the reaction that occurred previously. Thus it is directed towards maintenance and educational-type activities. Some of the interventions are very similar to those which arise at the primary level but they occur after, rather than before, a reaction has occurred.

As Neuman points out, the normal line of defence, or the individual's ability to respond to stressors after they have been affected and have already begun to react to stress, may be different from the beginning stage. In some instances it may settle at a lower level if the lines of defence have been permanently damaged. However in other cases, a 'higher level of wellness' can be achieved if the normal line of defence is strengthened and widened.

Knowledge and skills for practice

Since the emphasis of this model is on the interrelationship of all variables which affect human beings, the knowledge required is drawn from psychological, physiological, sociocultural and developmental theories, all of which can affect human behaviour. The focus is on identifying universal stressors (stressors which can affect anyone) and considering their impact in each of the four areas. Neuman and Young (1972) use loss as an example of a universal stressor which may lead to patient problems. They then clarify the knowledge required in each of the four areas. For example, theories about role, cultural change and social structure may be related to sociocultural loss. Similarly, theories about sensory deprivation, immune response and pain may be associated with physiological loss.

Another feature of this model is its emphasis on health promotion and illness prevention which leads to a necessity for knowledge and skills related to teaching and learning. If nurses wish to develop their ability as health educators, then this would become an essential component of the curriculum.

Similarly the health team approach which is advocated in the model leads to a requirement that nurses have an understanding of the structure and scope of the health care services and of the services that can be offered by different occupational groups.

It can be seen that the knowledge base required in order to be able to work with this model is very wide. However, Neuman (1972) suggests that the framework could be used to clarify different levels of nursing practice.

Assessment using the health care systems model

Neuman (1980) suggests that there are three basic principles to be considered in relationship to a nursing assessment. They are that:

- 'Good assessment requires knowledge of all the factors influencing a patient's perceptual field.
- The meaning that a stressor has to the patient is validated by the patient as well as by the care giver.
- Factors in the care giver's perceptual field that influence her assessment of the patient's situation should become apparent.'

Unlike some of the other models which have been described, the assessment format in this instance is fairly unstructured. However Neuman has identified a number of categories which must be included during assessment. They include:

- Biographical data.
- Stressors from the patient's perception — those factors which the patient sees as causing the major difficulties.
- Stressors from the nurse's perception — those factors which the nurse sees as causing the major difficulties.

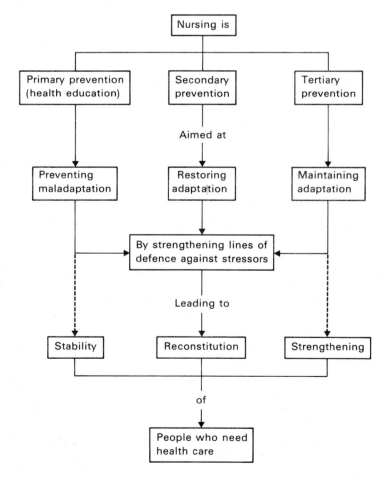

Fig. 8.2 *A diagrammatic representation of the health care systems model.*

- Intrapersonal, interpersonal and extrapersonal factors affecting an individual and his or her personal relationships. These are the responses to the stressors and may be considered under four categories, namely physiological, psychological, sociocultural and developmental factors.
- A statement of the problems in rank order reconciling any variation between the perceptions of the nurse and the perceptions of the patient.

During assessment Neuman suggests that a progressive approach is taken, moving from general points to more specific details. This is achieved through gaining initial information by general questions and observations and gradually progressing towards more specific assessment and categorisation of information.

In order to obtain the necessary information about stressors which are present, Neuman suggests that six basic questions should be posed and answered by both the patient and the nurse. In this way variations in perception can be identified so that they can be discussed and reconciled. The six questions, slightly modified for use in the United Kingdom, are:

1. What do you consider to be your major problem, difficulty or area of concern?

2. How has this affected your usual pattern of living or life style?

3. Have you ever experienced a similar problem previously? If so, what was that problem and how did you handle it? Was your handling of the problem successful?

4. What do you anticipate for yourself in the future as a consequence of your present situation?

5. What are you doing and what can you do to help yourself?

6. What do you expect care givers, family, friends and others to do for you?

As information is gathered, more specific questions may need to be asked within each category in order to ascertain more detailed information. By recording both the patient's and the nurse's responses to each question area, any variation in response can be identified and, whenever possible, reconciled. It must be remembered, however, that the client's perceptions and values must always be respected.

The categorisation of the data, once collected, does follow a more formal structure. It is classified into three major areas — intrapersonal, interpersonal and extrapersonal factors — and each case further subdivided into groups related to physiological, psychological and developmental factors. Neuman also emphasises that information may be gathered from other sources such as other health care workers or laboratory tests. A suggested format for recording data is shown in Figure 8.3.

Ward:	Admission Date:	Consultant:
		GP: Tel. No's:
		House Officer:
Age:	Marital Status:	Social Worker
DOB:	Occupation:	Relatives Staying:
Religion:	Baptised:	Relevant Past Medical History:
Likes to be Referred to as:		
NEXT OF KIN: Tel. No's: Name: Address:		
Meaningful Others:		
		Allergies/Infectious Diseases:
Dependents/Siblings:		
TYPE OF ADMISSION: Emergency/Waiting List:		
Medical Diagnosis:		
Reason for Admission:		Drugs Taken at Home:
Surgery/Treatment:		

Fig. 8.3 *The assessment form.*

Stressors

(A) What do you consider to be your major problem, difficulty or area of concern?

Patient's perception	Nurse's perception

(B) How has this affected your usual pattern of living or life-style?

Patient's perception	Nurse's perception

(C) Have you ever experienced a similar problem previously? If so, what was that problem and how did you handle it? Was it successful?

Patient's perception	Nurse's perception

(D) What do you anticipate for yourself in the future as a consequence of your present situation?

Patient's perception	Nurse's perception

(E) What are you doing and what can you do to help yourself?

Patient's perception	Nurse's perception

(F) What do you expect care givers, family, friends, or others to do for you?

Patient's perception	Nurse's perception

Summary

Intrapersonal

Interpersonal

Extrapersonal

Fig. 8.3 *The assessment form (contd.).*

Returning to Mr Smith and concentrating on his nutritional state, the responses given by both the patient and the nurses included:

Question 1

What do you consider to be your major problem, difficulty or area of concern?

Patient's perception Not able to look after myself and manage things how I like them.

Nurse's perception Independence reduced by restricted movement. Joints of fingers, hands and wrists severely affected by rheumatoid arthritis. Thin with loose clothes indicating weight loss.

Question 2

How has this affected your usual pattern of living or life style?

Patient's perception It has affected the timing of my meals and what is available. The ability to prepare meals or drinks by myself has been lost.

Nurse's perception Reduced food intake leading to weight loss. Dislike of food prepared by others.

Question 3

Have you ever experienced a similar problem previously? If so, what was that problem and how did you handle it? Was your handling of the problem successful?

Patient's perception No previous experience, although this has been coming on for years.

Nurse's perception Problem should have been identified earlier to prevent current situation.

Question 4

What do you anticipate for yourself in the future as a consequence of your present situation?

Patient's perception I hope to gain strength in hands and arms so that I can cook my own meals. I think that the physiotherapist will be able to help me.

Nurse's perception Hopes for full independence in preparing meals may be unrealistic. Occupational therapist may be able to advise on management.

Question 5

What are you doing and what can you do to help yourself?

Patient's perception I agreed to hospital admission reluctantly to try and get strength back.

Nurse's perception Unhappy about being in hospital and losing further independence but should be able to regain some aspects of self-care as is well motivated.

Question 6

What do you expect care givers, family, friends and others to do for you?

Patient's perception Neighbours already help with the garden, and the home help cleans, but it is unfair to expect them to do meals and anyway I don't like the food they cook. Meals-on-wheels food is always cold and awful, not like my own cooking.

Nurse's perception Dislikes receiving help from others. Unsuitable food often provided leading to inadequate dietary intake.

Summary

Intrapersonal

Physical Weight loss, insufficient food intake, reduced function from rheumatoid arthritis.

Psychosocial Hopes for full independence but is aware this may not be possible.

Developmental Is now aware that adjustments in life style are required because of physical disability.

Interpersonal

Physical Dislike of others cooking has contributed to poor nutritional intake.

Psychosocial Feels neighbours already contribute enough.

Developmental Network of supports small as no immediate family in district.

Extrapersonal

Physical Dislikes Meals-on-wheels. Food unsuitable.

Psychosocial No alternative services available locally.

Developmental Dependency may increase because of disease and aging processes. Needs to plan for the future.

Neuman includes problem identification as part of assessment and in Mr Smith's case both he and the nurse were able to agree on the difficulties listed below. Since none are immediately life-threatening, the priority was also agreed between the patient and nurse.

1. Loss of independence in preparing own meals.
2. Insufficient calorie intake to maintain weight.
3. Possibility of becoming more dependent in the future.

Neuman points out, however, that when this format is used, reassessment is a continuous process as the client's condition and perceptions alter and intervention is effective in reaching stated goals.

Care planning

The planning stage using this approach includes:

- A decision as to whether primary, secondary or tertiary action is required.
- A statement of goals and the rationale for them.
- A prescription.

Whenever possible, plans should be made for both immediate and future action although not all information would be available at the time of an initial assessment.

The goals of care may be directed towards preventing maladaptation, restoring adaptation or maintaining adaptation by either reducing the stresses or strengthening the lines of defence. While it would be hoped that a client can return to his or her previous level of wellness or even improve, this is not always the case and in Mr Smith's situation it would be unrealistic. So for him a new level which he finds acceptable may have to be sought. Figure 8.4 shows the goals.

Problem (i.e. response to stressor)	Goal (i.e. agreed adaptive behaviour)	
1. Loss of independence in preparing meals due to affects of rheumatoid arthritis	Able to make hot drinks and prepare light meals without aid	Strengthen lines of defence
2. Insufficient calorie intake to maintain weight	Maintain weight at present level	Remove stressor
3. Possibility of becoming more dependent in the future	Identify possible future sources of support	Strengthen lines of defence

Fig. 8.4 *The problem and goal statements.*

Actions for all three types of goals are included in the care plan but in different categories. Thus all are considered: primary action, aimed at anticipating difficulties before they arise in order to reduce or remove them; secondary action aimed at restoring health; and tertiary action aimed at maintaining health. Figure 8.5 shows Mr Smith's plan.

Primary action	Secondary action	Tertiary action
1.	1. Refer to occupational therapist for assessment, provision of aids and teaching use of aids.	1. Arrange home assessment with occupational therapist.
	2. Provide opportunities to practise once every day in ward kitchen.	2. Draw up a menu plan with Mr Smith for light meals.
2.	Discuss food values with Mr Smith and help with menu choice. Provide intake of at least 1500 calories per day. If hospital menu unsuitable ask dietician to visit.	Teach Mr Smith to plan his own diet within limits of ability in order to maintain his weight.
3. Identify local support system available to Mr Smith. Discuss possible attendance at local disabled dining clubs.		

Fig. 8.5 *The nursing action.*

Neuman emphasises that as care progresses, the situation may alter. During evaluation the actual outcomes of care are reviewed and compared with the stated ones. It may be necessary to revise any of the four steps of the process. In other words, further assessment may be required; the goals may need to be reconsidered; the action may need to be adjusted; or the time span allowed for change readjusted.

A patient care study

The assessment and care plan shown below are for a 40 year old woman, Mrs Dorothy Baxter, who has just been admitted to hospital to undergo a planned abdominal hysterectomy.

As suggested in the model, biographical data is collected in a fairly standard fashion followed by a semi-structured interview and a summary of the information. Emphasis is placed on the shared understanding between the nurse and the patient of the circumstances. The assessment focuses on identifying actual or potential stressors and their effects at an intrapersonal, interpersonal and extrapersonal level as well as the current strength of the lines of defence. Figure 8.6 shows the information recorded following Mrs Baxter's initial assessment.

Ward: *Neuman* Admission Date: *27.2.85*		Consultant: *Mr Tindle*
Mrs Dorothy Baxter *57 The Beeches* *High Town*		GP: *Dr Hardwick* Tel. No's: *66531*
		House Officer: *Dr Jamieson*
Age: *40*	Marital Status: *Married*	Social Worker *None*
DOB: *30·11·44*	Occupation: *Housewife*	Relatives Staying: *No*
Religion: *C of E*	Baptised:	Relevant Past Medical History:
Likes to be Referred to as: *Dotty*		*No serious illness.* *Dilatation and curettage* *on 15·12·84.* *Heavy bleeding for 18 months.*
NEXT OF KIN: *Husband* Tel. No's: *67841* Name: *Mr G Baxter* Address: *As above*		
Meaningful Others: *Mrs Agnes Bones (sister)* *43 The Elms, High Town* *Tel. 61847*		Allergies/Infectious Diseases: *Shellfish*
Dependents/Siblings: *3 children* *Peter (18) - at university* *James (16) + Sally (13) - at home*		
TYPE OF ADMISSION: Emergency/Waiting List: *Waiting list*		
Medical Diagnosis: *Menorrhagia due to fibroids.*		
Reason for Admission: *For abdominal hysterectomy.*		Drugs Taken at Home: *Iron tablet - 1 daily.* *Paracetamol for headaches.*
Surgery/Treatment:		

Fig. 8.6 *The initial assessment.*

STRESSORS

a. What do you consider to be your major problem, difficulty or area of concern?

Patient's perception:
The pain with my periods and very heavy bleeding. It got so bad that I couldn't cope with looking after my family. I'd bleed for 3 weeks every month.

Care giver's perception:
Menorrhagia. Anaemia. Looks tired and anxious.

b. How has this affected your usual pattern of living or life-style?

Patient's perception:
Find it difficult to run the house. Don't go out because of the risk of 'flooding'. Irritable with the children. Tired all the time. Affects my relationship with my husband.

Care giver's perception:
Lethargy and tiredness. Irritable. Restricted social and personal activities.

c. Have you ever experienced a similar problem previously? If so, what was that problem and how did you handle it? Was it successful?

Patient's perception:
Had a D&C 3 months ago so at least I know about hospitals and am not bothered about operation. My mother came to cope with the children so arrangements worked well but I do miss them and worry that they will be alright.

Care giver's perception:
Good insight into hospital care. Home arrangements well organised. Concerned about missing the family.

d. What do you anticipate for yourself in the future as a consequence of your present situation?

Patient's perception:
Relief from pain and bleeding. Return to my normal self in next to no time. I know I'll have to take it easy and not lift things for a while but I heal very quickly. I don't expect the operation will be very different from the D&C.

Care giver's perception:
Has slightly unrealistic expectations of speed of recovery. Limited understanding of current surgery.

e. What are you doing and what can you do to help yourself?

Patient's perception:
Can look after myself independently at the moment. I take iron tablets and Panadol for the pain. Warm baths seem to help too. I like being independent.

Care giver's perception:
Will need help immediately postoperatively with daily living activities. May find it difficult to depend upon the nurses immediately postoperatively.

Fig. 8.7 The in-depth assessment.

f. What do you expect care givers, family, friends or others to do for you?

Patient's perception:
Mother will stay as long as necessary at home. My husband really wants me back to my old self. I'm sure the nurses and doctors will look after me when I'm here but I won't need anyone else at home.

Care giver's perception:
Good family support. Husband more anxious than he has admitted to his wife. May need some help for a short while after discharge from hospital.

Summary
Intrapersonal factors
Physical:
Menorrhagia, lethargy and tiredness from anaemia.

Psychosociocultural:
Is optimistic about outcome of care.

Developmental:
Feels secure in her role in the family and wishes to be able to return to full participation.

Interpersonal factors

Physical:
Is unable to look after family fully.
Symptoms have limited her physical relationship with husband.

Psychosociocultural:
Social activities limited due to heavy bleeding and tiredness.

Developmental:
Family are sufficiently independent to support through period of operation and recovery.

Extrapersonal

Physical:
Needs are cared for at present.

Psychosociocultural:
No financial or occupational difficulties. Has a supportive family.

Developmental:
No concern about loss of reproductive ability.

Fig. 8.7 The in-depth assessment (contd.).

From the information gathered, Mrs Baxter and the nurse can reconcile any variances that they have. For instance, Mrs Baxter may have slightly unrealistic hopes about her rate of recovery and will need to discuss how quickly she will be able to return to her usual 'level of wellness' (Question D). Similarly because of her fondness of independence, particular attention may need to be paid to the way in which the immediate postoperative period is dealt with as at that time she will lose some of her independence and require support from the nurses. These situations have been recognised within the care plan seen in Figure 8.8 where problems 1 and 5 have been recognised in order to increase Mrs Baxter's understanding, thus hoping to strengthen her own lines of defence.

The goal of problem 4, lethargy due to anaemia, is concerned with the removal of a stressor.

The care which is aimed towards preventing complications is considered under primary intervention. Thus the preoperative measures taken to reduce the risks of complications occurring are recorded in this section, shown in problem 5.

Intervention to restore health is recorded under secondary treatment. This is problem 2, where anxiety already exists about family separation; the purpose is to plan intervention to reduce the stressor.

In line with Neuman's recommendations, tertiary care is planned early in the procedure. It is aimed at maintaining health in the future. Thus discharge plans (associated with problem 1) and management of diet to reduce the risks of anaemia are incorporated in this section. Other items may become apparent as Mrs Baxter progresses through her hospital stay and can be added at any time.

The health care systems approach offers an alternative approach to nursing which many nurses may enjoy. It is very broad in its approach, using theories from several fields, but it offers a flexible framework which can be easily adjusted to many fields of nursing work. Although at first sight the framework for assessment may seem to be too vague, with skilled use the amount of information obtained can be great, and the approach ensures that the patient's own perception of his condition is not overriden by that of the health care worker.

Problems	Goals	Primary Treatment (prevention)	Secondary Treatment (intervention)	Tertiary Treatment (follow up)
1. Limited knowledge about details and outcome of impending surgery.	a) Can explain surgery & care while in hospital. b) Is realistic about length of time required for convalescence.		a) Explain surgery using diagrams. b) Give details of pre and post-op care. c) Discuss arrangements for returning home.	a) Arrange discharge date with patient and family. Discuss rate of return to normal. Check home support for 2 weeks after discharge.
2. Slightly anxious about separation from family.	Can keep in contact with family member at least once a day.		Discuss visiting arrangements with family. Allow free access. Explain phoning procedures.	
3. Anxious about heavy bleeding preoperatively.	Bleeding will be contained by pads.		Give supply of pads in locker. Provide disposal bags. Situate bed near toilet.	
4. Lethargy due to anaemia.	Patient can fulfil activities of daily living without feeling over-tired.		Explain cause of lethargy. Explain and supervise pre-op blood transfusion. 1/2 hrly pulse, hrly BP and T while transfusion in progress.	Explain dietary factors related to iron sources.
5. Impending surgery leading to risks of: a) respiratory distress. b) nausea + vomiting.	Respiratory rate between 1-20. No cough or sputum. No nausea or vomiting post-operatively.	Pre-op visit by physio. 10 deep breaths/hour as soon as alert post-op. NBM from 7 a.m. 28.2.85. Give anti-emetic with analgesic post-op.		

Problems	Goals	Primary Treatment (prevention)	Secondary Treatment (intervention)	Tertiary Treatment (follow up)
c) Pain	Pain score of 5 or less on Painometer by 2nd day Post-operatively.	Explain pain levels and use of painometer pre-operatively.	Check Pain levels 2 hourly on even hour. Give analgesic if score higher than 4, following prescription.	
d) Deep vein thrombosis	Calf soft and pain free.	Fit elastic stockings. Teach ankle exercises. Advise not to cross legs. Discuss advantages of early mobilisation.	Check calves daily at 10 a.m. Supervise exercises as soon as alert post-op. Leave stockings in situ except for hygiene until fully mobile.	
e) Infection	Maintain temperature of 37°C or less.		Record temperature 6hrly for at least 48 hours or until stable for 4 consecutive readings. Check wound for inflammation and for dis-	
			charge daily at time of bath.	
f) Shock	BP 120/80 mmHg P 84/min		Record BP and pulse hourly for 6 hours post-operatively. Then reduce to 4 hourly if stable.	

Fig. 8.8 The care plan.

9 | An Interaction Model for Nursing

A number of models based on the theory of symbolic interaction have been developed for nursing. The model proposed by King, an eminent American nurse, focuses on interaction, and has been applied by many American nursing teams. It uses concepts which King found to be repeatedly occurring in nursing literature, research, teaching and practice. The model was developed through a research project. In the research study, all the interactions between nurses and patients were observed in two different settings from admission to discharge. One group consisted of patients admitted to hospital for surgical procedures, and the other, of patients admitted to hospital in an acute crisis, for example, myocardial infarction. The study set out to answer the following questions:

- What is the nursing act?
- What is the nursing process?
- What is the goal of nursing?
- Who are nurses and how are they educated to practise?
- How and where is nursing practised?
- Who needs nursing in society?

The result of the study was to confirm King's assumptions about the nature of nursing, and led to the development of the model. King's basic concept of nursing sees it as a process which involves action, reaction, interaction and transaction. Through this process, nursing assists individuals of any age and background to meet basic needs in carrying out the acts of daily living and to cope with health and illness at a specific point in the life cycle (King, 1971).

Four universal concepts form the basis of the model: social systems, health, perception and interpersonal relationships. King believes these four concepts apply to any individual, and that they represent a conceptual base for nursing practice. The universal concepts are linked together through the process of interaction. People live and grow in a social system through relating to others who are part of that social system. These interpersonal relationships occur according to the individual's perceptions; and individual perceptions influence life and health.

Social systems Social systems exist wherever there are people living. Within them, individuals develop social relationships and form groups to achieve common goals. The social system guides interaction betweeen individuals, social relationships, the setting of rules of behaviour and modes of action taken. Beliefs, attitudes, values and customs are all learned within social systems. Examples of social systems are the family, the school and the church, and each shares the common characteristic of having an observable structure — roles for people to occupy, status awarded to such roles, obvious authority, and rules of behaviour. Every individual is part of a number of social systems and these together make up the network of social systems which influence life and health. For example, the individual's membership of a specific family, racial group and church, together influences behaviour and beliefs. It will lead to some relationships being seen as good, and others as bad, and to certain judgements and decisions being made. People who grow up in a family with liberal views, who accept a wide range of people into their sphere of friendship, and who believe that everyone has the right to be happy will have different beliefs and values from those whose family is tightly knit and introverted and who value rigid rules of behaviour.

Perception Perception is the individual's representation of reality — that is, objects, people and events. Perception varies from one individual to another and is dependent upon past experience, background, knowledge and emotional state. It is also influenced by the person's social systems network, and in turn, affects interpersonal relationships.

Interpersonal relationships This is interaction between two or more people, and is therefore a meeting of different expectations, goals, needs and values. Interaction always involves action, as action is interpreted as exerting some control and holding some responsibility for events that transpire. For example, when two people meet, both act to control what happens between them and are responsible for the result. If neither speaks, and the interaction ends by both turning away from each other, it is because of the non-speaking act. Both involved are responsible for the result.

Health King sees health as related to coping with stress. Her model is holistic in its concerns, encompassing the physical, emotional and social components of people. In her words it 'relates to the way in which the individual deals with the stress of growth and development while functioning within a cultural pattern in which he was born or to which he attempts to conform' (King, 1971).

King believes that health has different meanings for individuals and groups in different cultures, and often for individuals within the same culture. The medical model of health and illness contrasts sharply with that of the sociologists, and nurses who have a major input in helping individuals during life crises need to understand the different perceptions of clients to these two models.

King's model is based on these four universal concepts of social systems, perception, interpersonal relationships and health, and on nursing as essentially an interactive process.

Beliefs and values

People are seen as functioning in social systems, through interpersonal relationships. Such relationships occur according to peoples' perceptions, which in turn influence their lives and health. Thus, the social systems are the framework of living, interpersonal relationships are the processes in which people engage in during living, and these processes are determined by perceptions and health. Throughout life, people:

1. Are reactive beings. Individuals react to situations, persons and objects as they perceive them.

2. Are time-orientated beings. The present is based on what has happened in the past, and perceptions of what is happening now influence predictions for the future.

3. Are social beings. They like being with others, and life focuses on social living. People behave sometimes in a similar, and often in a dissimilar fashion to others as they interact with them by verbal and non-verbal actions. Interaction takes place with people and things in the immediate environment and social systems which surround them. People adapt to life and health under the influence of internal and external environmental factors. Adaptation arises out of interaction in social relationships.

The goals of nursing

The overall goal of nursing is to help people and groups to attain, maintain, and restore health. When the goal of life and health cannot be achieved, such as in the terminally ill, then nurses give care and help individuals to die with dignity.

Nursing aims at the achievement of health in individuals by meeting three basic health needs. These needs are:

1. The need for usable health information at a time when individuals need it and are able to use it.

2. The need for preventive care to prevent ill health.

3. The need for care when ill.

The specific sub-goal to be achieved by nurses in order to meet these health needs is to establish transactions between themselves and clients, their families and other social systems.

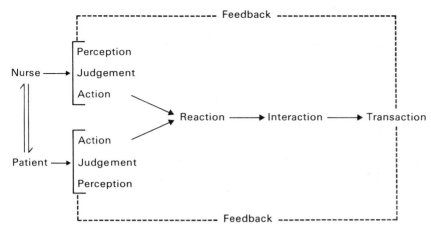

Fig. 9.1 *The observable nursing process (after King, 1971).*

Knowledge and skills for practice

Nursing is seen as a helping activity which provides a service which meets a social need. Its service provides care to individuals and groups who are ill, and it promotes health through education. The knowledge base therefore revolves around the four universal concepts — social systems, perception, interpersonal relations and health — and about the physiology, psychology and sociology of the human state. Nurses require specific skills of observation and communication to collect information, to make decisions and to implement a plan of care based on problems amenable to nursing action. Technical skills are seen as an essential part of practice in gathering reliable data about physiological parameters of the health state.

The nursing process consists of action, reaction, interaction and transaction. (See Figure 9.1.) Basing practice on the knowledge and skills already mentioned, the nurse needs to become skilled in this interactive process before effective professional practice can be achieved.

Action

Whenever two people meet, some kind of action is involved. It is a sequence of behaviours or activities which includes:

- Recognising presenting conditions.
- Doing something related to the condition or situation.
- Motivation to do something to achieve desired goals.

For example, the nurse may decide, with the patient, to try to walk him or her from bed to chair. To do this, and following on from it, interaction occurs.

Reaction

This is simply the result of the action and interaction. How did the patient react to the suggestion of walking? How did the patient react when walking? Reaction is the feedback received after taking action, through interaction.

Interaction

This is an interplay of communication between two or more people. In nursing, it always involves the nurse and patient, but may include others. In the walking example, the nurse and patient interact in carrying out the action.

Transaction

This is reaching some agreement to pursue an action plan to achieve the desired outcome.

Nursing skills and knowledge are channelled towards helping people through the interactive process, which forms the fundamental nursing expertise available to help people to become healthy. Figure 9.2 is a diagrammatic representation of King's model.

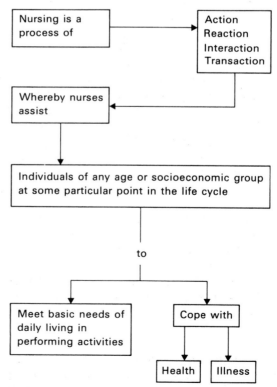

Fig. 9.2 *A diagrammatic representation of King's interaction model (after NDCG, 1973).*

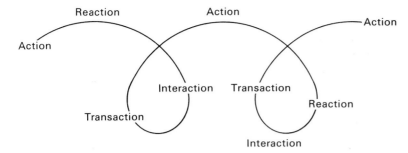

Fig. 9.3 *The continuous interactive process of nursing.*

Assessment using an interaction model

The stages of the nursing process are highly integrated in the model described by King, and relate to the interactive process of action — interaction — reaction — transaction. The steps are circular and occur continuously as nursing takes place. (See Figure 9.3.) These four universal concepts can be used as the basic framework in assessment.

Social Systems Through interaction, the nurse and patient establish the social system network related to the presenting situation. This includes present and past social systems included in the patient's life. In the care of Mr Smith, the nurse, in exploring the problem of weight loss, notes that he lives alone within a geographic group of people — his neighbours — who are polite to each other, and help out in acts such as gardening, but who have little personal closeness. He has no family, having lost his wife 20 years ago, and he values his role as an autonomous independent being. Because of his past experiences with social systems, it is acceptable to him for neighbours and home helps to keep his home and garden tidy but it is unacceptable for them to carry out personal services such as providing meals.

Perception The patient's perception of himself, his world and his current state are fundamental to effective nursing in this model. Together, the nurse and patient interact to establish how the current position is viewed and the hopes the patient has for the future. The perception of Mr Smith towards his own personal predicament revealed his reality which saw others as being 'put upon' in supporting him and in his expectation to achieve relative independence in the future.

Interpersonal relationships Assessment of this universal concept involves both the relationship between the nurse and patient and relationships with others. It is inextricably linked with the previous two concepts and involves feelings about others, as well as the behaviour of relating to people. The quality and extent of relationships concerned in the case of Mr Smith could only be superficially considered in the early stages of assessment, but they develop as the nurse and patient interact.

Health Health assessment involves getting information from the patient and professionals involved to identify stresses and the ability to agree that they exist. These may include potential or actual stresses which promote ill health. Rheumatoid arthritis, pain, loss of movement, loss of weight and loss of appetite were all identified as barriers to health in the assessment of Mr Smith.

The organisation of information in assessment, using the model described by King, is based on these four universal concepts. In some practice teams, an open assessment form with these concepts as headings may be appropriate. An example of a more structured approach is in Figure 9.4. It focusses on assessment of the 14 activities of daily living described by Henderson (1966), in relation to King's 4 universal concepts. Assessment is perception and action, and problems are identified through reaction and interaction. Transaction leads to the formulation of a care plan and its implementation.

Evaluating care involves the whole interactive process again, as does any reassessment and replanning.

For example, the extract from a care plan in Figure 9.5 could only be constructed after the whole of the interactive process has been completed. But the process begins again when the nurse gives the analgesics and milk drink (action and interaction); observes the patient and later seeks his opinion to establish the effectiveness of the strategy (reaction); and decides to continue with the plan or to revise it (transaction).

Problem	Goal	Action
Unable to sleep more than 2 hours at night because of pain in nose.	Will sleep for at least 6 hours for 3 nights in succession.	1. Give hot milky Ovaltine with analgesics prescribed when patient asks for it. 2. Patient can watch television until feels sleepy.

Fig. 9.5 *A care plan item.*

Care planning

The care plan is both a statement of the transaction agreed upon by the nurse and patient and a guide to the nature of the interactive process to be engaged in while nursing takes place. It is a prescription for action; a means by which to judge reaction; an account of planned interaction. Once transactions are agreed upon, specific

Date of admission:	Date of assessment:	Nurse:

MALE ___ AGE SURNAME . . . . FORENAMES . . . .

FEMALE ___ DATE OF BIRTH . . . . Prefers to be addressed as

. . . .

ADDRESS OF USUAL RESIDENCE

TYPE OF ACCOMMODATION

FAMILY/OTHERS AT THIS RESIDENCE

NEXT OF KIN | NAME | ADDRESS

| RELATIONSHIP | TEL. NO.

SIGNIFICANT OTHERS

SUPPORT SERVICES

SIGNIFICANT LIFE CRISIS

REASON FOR ADMISSION

MEDICAL INFORMATION (e.g. diagnosis, past history, allergies) | WEIGHT _____

URINE

TEMP.   PULSE
BP   RESP.

DISCHARGE ARRANGEMENTS: (to be completed on admission)

MAIN SOURCE FOR ASSESSMENT: | PROJECTED DATE OF DISCHARGE:

SIGNIFICANT OTHERS INTERVIEWED: YES/NO

IF YES? DETAILS OF INTERVIEW | ARRANGEMENTS DISCUSSED WITH
RELATIVES: _____ OTHERS ___

HOME HELP _____

D/N
H/V

Fig. 9.4 *The assessment form.*

ADL	SOCIAL SYSTEMS	PERCEPTION	INTERPERSONAL RELATIONS	HEALTH STATE AND USUAL PHYSICAL CAPABILITIES
BREATHING				
EATING AND DRINKING				
ELIMINATING				
MOVEMENT AND POSTURE				
SLEEP AND REST				
DRESS AND UNDRESS				
BODY TEMPERATURE				

ADL	SOCIAL SYSTEMS	PERCEPTION	INTERPERSONAL RELATIONS	HEALTH STATE AND USUAL PHYSICAL CAPABILITIES
SKIN AND PERSONAL HYGIENE				
AVOID DANGER IN ENVIRONMENT				
COMMUNICATION				
RELIGIOUS MATTERS				
WORK				
PLAY				
LEARNING				

Fig. 9.4 *The assessment form (contd.).*

goals are set in order to give direction and to be used as a yardstick in determining reaction — or in other words to evaluate. The specific goals must relate realistically to the goals implicit in the model. The specific goals must establish transactions between the nurse and patient:

- To attain health.
- To maintain health.
- To restore health.
- To give dignified care.

Thus the overall goal of this model is holistic health. The goal statements should, as well as being assessable for evaluation purposes, be formulated by the nurse and patient and represent a transaction. (See Figure 9.6.)

Problem (i.e. reaction and interaction)	Goal (i.e. transaction)
1. Losing weight.	Will gain weight or remain same weight.
2. Unappy about home help and Meals-on-wheels providing food.	An alternative way of serving a cooked meal will be agreed upon.
3. Would like and feels will eventually be able to cook meal everyday.	Will be able to cook a meal independently.
4. Wants to remain in role of independent adult but not sure if this is possible.	Will be able to specifically say what he can be independent in, and what he is likely to be dependent in.

Fig. 9.6 *The problem and goal statement.*

In this example, nursing has aimed at restoring and maintaining those aspects of Mr Smith's life which he is concerned about and which affect his health.

Evaluation of the care given can be carried out by interaction with Mr Smith to see whether the stated goals have been achieved or not achieved or whether, in fact, there has been no movement in either of these directions.

The nursing action is written in terms of how the patient and nurse will work together to meet the goals. (See Figure 9.7.)

A patient care study

Mr Ted Donnelly has been admitted to the medical ward of a District General Hospital with acute bronchopneumonia. The initial action of his primary nurse was to record biographical data, and to interact with Mr Donnelly to obtain information about the 14 activities of daily living in the context of the 4 universal concepts.

Nursing Action

(i.e. action, reaction, interaction and transaction)

1. Discuss and plan daily intake of at least 1500 calories over next 24 hours — each day at 10 a.m.

2. Alternative way of providing a meal each day will be discussed when daily dietary plan is formulated.

3. Refer to occupational therapist for assessment, provision of aids and teaching.

4. Review current state of dependence each day.

Fig. 9.7 *The nursing action.*

The recordings that were made are noted in Figure 9.8.

From this information, the nurse was able to review needs related to:

- The giving of information about health.
- The prevention of ill health.
- The need for care.

She was then able to identify problems in the performance of the activities of daily living related to the patient's social systems network, perception, interpersonal relationships and health. In this case, the effects of the past and of the patient's attitudes and values had implications for the care to be given. The care is outlined in the care plan. (See Figure 9.9.)

The focus of the care plan is on the achievement of health through helping the patient to further develop interpersonal relationships with his social systems network, and to take into account his own perceptions of his predicament.

The productive cough (problem 1) and the associated feeling of being dirty (problem 3) were considered in the context of Mr Donnelly's usual social systems — his family, his social peers and his friends — and his interpersonal relations with his wife, as well in its reality as a physical symptom related to health.

Problems 2 and 4 had both health and interactive components, while problem 5, a feeling of isolation, was largely psychosocial.

Thus, the focus of the assessment and the care plan was on the patient as an interactive being, viewed within the context of his interaction with others.

Throughout this brief account of Mr Donnelly's care, the interactive process is emphasised. Nursing itself is seen as an interactive activity and the patient is seen as an interactive being. An interaction model emphasises this process and King sees it as the overriding concern of nursing.

Date of admission: 8·9·86	Date of assessment: 8·9·86	Nurse: *Brenda Miles*
MALE __X__ AGE 51 SURNAME *Donnelly* .. FORENAMES *Edward William*		
FEMALE ___ DATE OF BIRTH ...*7·8·36*......... Prefers to be addressed as *Ted*		

ADDRESS OF USUAL RESIDENCE	*Highway House, High Street, Biggan Village*
TYPE OF ACCOMMODATION	*Detached house – 4 bedrooms, bathroom and toilet on both levels. Central heating.*
FAMILY/OTHERS AT THIS RESIDENCE	*Wife*
NEXT OF KIN	NAME ADDRESS *Fiona Donnelly As above* RELATIONSHIP TEL. NO. *38198*
SIGNIFICANT OTHERS	*Daughter – married with two children, lives in S. Africa.*
SUPPORT SERVICES	*Housekeeper*
SIGNIFICANT LIFE CRISIS	*When he had to give up work – two years ago.*
REASON FOR ADMISSION	*Acute bronchopneumonia*

MEDICAL INFORMATION (e.g. diagnosis, past history, allergies) *Cor pulmonale since 1983* *(3 years)*	WEIGHT *12st 4lbs* URINE *NAD, SG 1006* TEMP. *39.8°C* PULSE *98/min* BP *160/90* RESP. *36/min* *mm Hg*
MAIN SOURCE FOR ASSESSMENT: *Ted*	DISCHARGE ARRANGEMENTS: (to be completed on admission) *To be discharged home when medical problem resolved.* PROJECTED DATE OF DISCHARGE: *? 15·9·86*
SIGNIFICANT OTHERS INTERVIEWED: YES/NO IF YES? DETAILS OF INTERVIEW	ARRANGEMENTS DISCUSSED WITH RELATIVES: ____ OTHERS ___ HOME HELP _____ D/N H/V

Fig. 9.8 *The assessment.*

ADL	SOCIAL SYSTEMS	PERCEPTION	INTERPERSONAL RELATIONS	HEALTH STATE AND USUAL PHYSICAL CAPABILITIES
BREATHING	Ashamed of coughing up sputum - feels dirty.	"My cough is worse. I'd give anything for a new pair of lungs."	Conscious that noisy breathing and cough "make it difficult for people - "my wife must find me repulsive".	Very "short of breath" - unable to take more than 20 steps. Coughing up large amounts of sputum.
EATING AND DRINKING	Wife prepares food. Main meal at noon. Likes plain food.	"I eat well." Likes all foods. Drinks tea - whisky at night.		Slightly overweight. Well hydrated.
ELIMINATING	Hates using bedpan or commode.	Is aware of other people noticing odour from elimination.	Embarassed by need to discuss elimination with others.	Opens bowels daily. Urinalysis-NAD. Does not wake up at night to pass urine.
MOVEMENT AND POSTURE	Restricted in attending valued activities- e.g. golf club.	"Can't do as much as I could because of the breathing."		Can walk slowly from bed to day room and up-stairs. But breathless in doing so.
SLEEP AND REST		"Sleep all the time."		Bed at 10 p.m., up at 6 a.m. Snoozes in morning and afternoon.
DRESS AND UNDRESS		"I don't bother much about appearances as long as I am warm."	"My wife gets annoyed if I don't get dressed during the day."	Independent in dressing.
BODY TEMPERATURE	No difficulty in keeping house warm.			

Fig. 9.8 The assessment (contd.).

ADL	SOCIAL SYSTEMS	PERCEPTION	INTERPERSONAL RELATIONS	HEALTH STATE AND USUAL PHYSICAL CAPABILITIES
SKIN AND PERSONAL HYGIENE	No outside assistance at home.	Feels dirty because unable to bathe without help.		
AVOID DANGER IN ENVIRONMENT				Socially isolated.
COMMUNICATION	Limited contact with friends because of poor mobility.	"I miss my nights in the pub."	"I get bad tempered with Fiona because I don't see anyone else."	
RELIGIOUS MATTERS	No formal religious practice.			
WORK	Retired Town Hall clerk. Retired early due to ill health.	"I feel useless and unable to do anything anymore."	Lost touch with friends. Relationship with wife strained through lack of outside stimulation.	Watches TV. Reads Daily Telegraph. No longer able to contribute to household activities.
PLAY	Used to play golf and go to pub 3x week. Gave up golf 3 years ago.			
LEARNING			"I'm too old to change my ways now."	Resistent to changing life style.

Fig. 9.8 The assessment (contd.).

DATE	NO.	PROBLEM	GOAL	NURSING ACTION	REVIEW DATE
		Basic need profile-			
8.9.86		Change in usual daily living circumstances	Maintain usual living pattern		
	1.	Productive cough	Will be able to cough up sputum easily and privately.	a. Provide a single room when available. b. Sputum mug in easy reach. c. Change sputum mug at 10 a.m., 2 p.m., 6 p.m., 10 p.m. d. Refer to physiotherapist	
	2.	Unable to walk far without becoming breathless. Embarassed about possibility of not reaching toilet.	Will go to toilet unaided without becoming distressed.	a. Put bed close to toilets. b. Provide urinal.	
	3.	Feels "dirty" about cough.	Will express such anxieties openly to nurses.	a. Signify aware- ness of his feelings whenever possible. b. Offer listening time when possible.	

NAME		NO.	PRIMARY NURSE
Mr Ted Donnelly		64	Brenda Miles

Fig. 9.9 The care plan.

DATE	NO.	PROBLEM	GOAL	NURSING ACTION	REVIEW DATE
	4.	Unable to bathe unaided.	Skin will be clean.	a. General bath with help of 2 nurses – Mon. and Thurs. mornings. b. Offer wash bowel at waking and before resting.	
	5.	Feels socially isolated because of immobility and feelings of being dirty.	Will express a desire to increase social activity.	a. Offer information about self-help group for patients with chronic obstructive airways disease. b. Introduce him to patients in similar situation. c. Discuss possibility of social activities for the future.	

NAME		NO.	PRIMARY NURSE
Mr Ted Donnelly		64	Brenda Miles

Fig. 9.9 *The care plan (contd.).*

10 | A Developmental Model for Nursing

Hildegard Peplau was one of the earliest American theorists to recognise and respond to the need for changes in nursing practice, and her particular area of interest was psychiatry. Her work dates back to the early fifties when, using a developmental framework, she published her thoughts in the book *Interpersonal relations in nursing* (1952). However, in line with her own beliefs, the views she presented then have, in themselves, continued to develop and grow as new knowledge has become available. Growth has occurred both through looking at small aspects of the model in greater depth and by giving fuller explanations to the unity of the whole model. Although her views were written primarily for psychiatric nurses, much of what she has to say can be of use to those working in other fields.

Peplau's work has been described as being influential in creating what is known as second order change, that is in influencing the system of nursing itself. In line with the arguments presented earlier for model-based practice, 'her ideas have provided an architectural design for the practice of a discipline' (Sills, 1978).

The need for a theoretical basis for practice is further emphasised by Peplau's views about professional accountability. She argues that this is not a new concept but one which has always been present in one guise or another, its purpose being to 'prod the professional towards proper behaviour in health care work' (1980). Originally it was masked in a dedication to duty, an expectation that individuals were committed to the service they offered with total devotion. As time has passed this concept has become outmoded and self-sacrifice and commitment are no longer acceptable in isolation. Questions are being asked such as 'What is it that nurses actually do? What is the specific service they offer? What are the health problems they can treat?' Initially these questions arose from the controlling bodies of an occupational group. While this still holds true and each nurse may be asked to account for her actions to her controlling organisation, Peplau sees some limitations in this system alone. She describes it as one which creates 'guilty knowledge' — knowledge of practice or malpractice which is not disclosed to the public. Social forces are such that there has been further growth in professional accountability, the practitioner being asked to account not only to a professional body but also, and maybe more importantly, to the public.

Peplau also stresses the need for accountability to oneself, a personal integrity in being honest about one's actions and being able to justify them. Thus there is a requirement for all nurses to constantly update the knowledge base from which they practise, to keep pace with new information, and to be prepared to revise theories.

Peplau argues that the care that a client *needs* may well be different from the care that a client *wants*. She suggests that if nurses only respond to what a client wants, they are at risk of providing nothing more than custodial care, consumer services or assistance to other health care workers. Therefore, clarity in the services offered by nursing and constant updating of knowledge and revision of theory are essential.

Beliefs and values

The emphasis of Peplau's approach is on the growth of both the patient and the nurse, stressing the phases and roles through which they both pass in the interpersonal process. The movement through phases follows a developmental pattern and leads to the growth of those concerned. She sees all individuals as unique people with both biological and psychological components who are capable of achieving new learning and making positive changes. As people are subjected to stress, so tension is created. In its turn tension creates energy, and this energy can either be well used, leading to growth, or poorly used, leading to regression. The response to the stress is dependent on its degree and the individual's ability to respond. This in turn is based on the stage of development and past experience of the individual concerned and will be different in every case. (See Figure 10.1.)

Peplau also recognises that all people have needs which need to be met. Thus a physical need may be for food or shelter and a psychological need may be for recognition or sharing. When needs are not met, growth of the individual will be inhibited. The presence of needs creates tension and, if needs continue to be unmet, frustra-

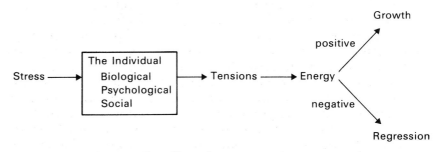

Fig. 10.1 *The effect of stress on an individual.*

tion can occur. However individuals strive towards development and growth through learning positive behaviours. If positive behaviours are not achieved, then regression can occur. Since we all live in an unstable environment, we are constantly faced with new situations, new problems to solve, and new experiences. Thus we continually have the opportunity to carry on developing throughout our life span.

The goals of nursing

Peplau views nursing in itself as a therapeutic interpersonal process involving a professional closeness or one-way interest in what is happening to another person. She sees the purpose of this relationship as two-fold. First and of immediate concern is the survival of the organism. However, once this goal has been achieved, a second purpose of the service offered by nurses is to help individuals to understand their health problems and to learn from their experiences with them. Stresses cannot, and indeed should not, be avoided but nurses can help patients to use the stress situations as learning experiences through which they can acquire new patterns of behaviour and thus change.

Peplau (1969) points out that when individuals undergo stress

> . . . self-concern is almost the exclusive force. The task of the nurse is not to sympathise with this self-concern but rather to aid the patient to bring to bear — to develop through use — his competence for seeing and understanding his predicament.

By assisting people in recognising their own reactions and coping mechanisms, nurses can help them to develop a fuller understanding of themselves and through this to evolve a foresight which will help them to prevent, when possible, future recurrences of illnesses. Thus nursing goes beyond the mothering and technical aspects of care into the realms of health teaching and preventive services. The goal is concerned with helping individuals in a forward movement of personality. It is concerned with creativity. In achieving this end, Peplau stresses that it is not only the patient or client who will develop but also the nurse through her increased understanding of the effects of universal stressors on different unique individuals.

In more recent years, Peplau has expressed a further view about nursing. She sees it not only as an interpersonal process concerned with individual clients, but also as a strong social force. She suggests that there is a swing towards the idea of good health as a right, not just a privilege, with an emphasis on health maintenance. With this change, there is a requirement that nurses become actively involved in planning health care programmes and in setting policies at both local and national levels. Because of their wide and varied contact with people, they are in a position not only to care for the sick but also to make public their views on issues concerned with health care. Thus another goal of nursing can be identified, that of influencing social policy.

Knowledge and skills for practice

To Peplau, the essence of nursing is in the relationship between the nurse and the client. She suggests that nursing care occurs within such an interpersonal relationship. Thus in order to help patients to meet their own needs, nurses must first become aware of themselves, their personal needs and their personal reactions. By doing this, they can manage their own behaviour rather than that of the patient and use themselves as the stimulus or therapeutic agent to which the patients will respond and which will cause them to modify their behaviour. She points out the very real danger of nurses behaving in such a way as to meet their own personal needs through seeking patient approval. For instance, 'doing something for' a patient may give satisfaction to the nurse and gain thanks from the patient but not achieve movement towards a goal of development for the patient.

Peplau suggests that nurses must develop the skill of attaining professional closeness, an attribute only learned through professional schooling. She differentiates professional closeness from physical closeness, interpersonal intimacy, and pseudo-closeness. Physical closeness is concerned with the physical act of mothering and is a relatively easy behaviour to acquire. Interpersonal closeness is the two-way interpersonal exchange, usually between two peers, where thoughts and ideas about new experiences are shared together purposely for the benefit of both. Pseudo-closeness is the sympathetic response given in answer to a given situation. 'Isn't that awful' or 'I'm so sorry' are examples of this sort of behaviour. She sees a danger in this type of response since it may block further understanding. While there may appear to be a closeness, it is only superficial.

Professional closeness, in contrast, contains elements of physical closeness and interpersonal intimacy but goes beyond. The focus of attention is exclusively upon the client rather than on both participants, and a professional's behaviour is adjusted in order to meet the client's needs. It requires that nurses show interest, concern and competence in the client's situation but can still manage their own personal responses.

In order to achieve this end, Peplau suggests that it is the task of the school to help students to study and understand their own reactions to stressful or difficult situations such as disfigurement, unpleasant odours or pain, in order that they can control their own reactions. Without attaining this ability, there is a risk of:

- Over-involvement at a personal level.
- Under-involvement with an emphasis on the clinical or technical components of work.

• Avoidance of clients with difficult problems by allocating them to students or untrained staff.

Alternatively, professional closeness allows an intimate relationship with a patient to develop, focused on the patient's personal needs or frustrations and aimed towards growth of that particular individual.

The type of stimulus the nurse provides in this situation must be based on knowledge. Peplau suggests that this should be very broad based and drawn from both the behavioural and the physical sciences, and theories of nursing. Thus universal knowledge can be applied and adapted to unique individuals. She suggests that in each new situation, there is an opportunity for new learning for the nurse as she sees the different ways people react to universal situations. Peplau also suggests that if there is a mismatch between the nurse's current knowledge and a client's response, then the nurse will be guided as to what further knowledge is needed in order to develop personally or to consider further theories.

While Peplau lays emphasis on the interpersonal nature of nursing, she does not neglect the technical side and points out that nurses must also acquire skills necessary to perform procedures related to nursing. Figure 10.2 is a diagrammatic representation of Peplau's developmental model.

Assessment using a developmental model

In line with developmental theory, Peplau suggests that a patient moves through four phases in his movement towards health which correspond with the four phases of the nursing process.

The orientation phase — assessment

In this phase both the patient and the nurse learn the nature of the difficulty that the patient is experiencing and they develop a mutual trust. The orientation phase is the stage at which data is collected in order that problems can be identified. It may be very rapid or extend over a long period of time, according to the particular nature of the situation.

The identification phase — planning

The second stage is reached when the patient recognises that he or she is forming a relationship with the nurse and the nurse plans the appropriate intervention. Peplau lays emphasis on the fact that since nurses have expert knowledge about nursing, the responsibility lies with them rather than the patients to formulate plans and goals. Her concern about the possible differences between what patients want and what they need is highlighted and she recognises that the goals of the nurse and the patient may not be the same. Part

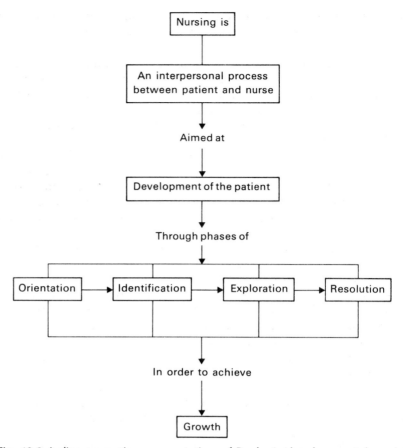

Fig. 10.2 *A diagrammatic representation of Peplau's developmental model.*

of the development of the relationship between them will be in the resolution of these variances, the nurse using expert knowledge in helping the patient to have a better understanding and insight into the particular health difficulty concerned.

The exploitation phase — implementation

At this stage of the patient's experience, there is recognition and response to the services that are offered by the nurse. The interpersonal process is fully utilised and both move towards mutually recognised goals. The nurse may act as counsellor, resource person, technician or take on any other appropriate role according to the situation.

The resolution phase — evaluation

As the health problem is overcome and the patient no longer requires a nursing service, so the ties that have grown between the nurse and the patient must be broken. The nurse evaluates the situation and learns from the experience in order to be able to apply new knowledge to further situations. The patient returns to an adult state of independence and freedom having hopefully grown.

Peplau suggests that there are two basic causes which may lead to a person seeking help from a health care worker when unwell. First, the individual concerned will have a 'felt need' — a problem that has arisen which requires a response. Second, the individual will have expectations of help from the professional person whose advice is sought. During the orientation or assessment phase, these needs and expectations are explored in order to clarify the situation. Peplau suggests that if emphasis at this stage is placed on the disease process and on ways in which it can be overcome, the emphasis of care will also be on the conquering of the disease. Alternatively if emphasis is placed on the personal growth of the individual, on considering the event which has led to a need for health care as a learning experience of life, then a more genuine consideration of the individual is likely to arise.

Because of the nature of Peplau's views, it would be inappropriate to follow a formal structure during the orientation or assessment phase of development, since the very essence of her approach is based on the relationship that is formed between the client and the nurse. It has been argued that the use of this model is confined to a limited number of clinical settings where the whole emphasis of care is based on the client's ability to recognise and accept the underlying cause of his or her difficulty. In areas where a greater emphasis is placed on achieving changes in current behaviour through other means, the approach may be considered as both time consuming and inappropriate.

Yet, with the current shift in emphasis towards the individual's rights in managing their own health, there is much to be learned from a model which lays emphasis on helping people to explore why they are facing difficulties. Without such information, the ability to manage in the future may be restricted. While the depth of such exploration can vary considerably, according to the particular situation or indeed the particular wishes of the client concerned, much can be learned by nurses in any setting from consideration of Peplau's views about personal development and growth.

Regardless of the unstructured approach to the assessment in this situation, it is still essential that information gathered during the orientation phase is recorded both for future reference and to assist in professional accountability.

Peplau does not describe or recommend a particular form of record keeping, but the method that we have used to apply the ideas behind her model of nursing is that of process recording using the SOAP format. The format uses the acronym SOAP to describe different stages of the process.

S This is the subjective experience as described by the client or patient. Direct quotes are often used. If the client is unable to contribute, it is quite acceptable to write 'none'.

O This is the objective observation that is made by the nurse. Such things as relevant laboratory findings may also be included in this section.

A This is the formal assessment or judgement made by nurses using both the subjective and objective data. It is the stage at which the information is analysed and at which the problems are identified.

P This is where a plan of action is decided upon, based on the problem identification and the subjective and objective data that has been gathered.

In some instances this format is extended to include the implementation and evaluation stages of the process. In this situation the following letters are added, making the acronym SOAPIER.

I The implementation stage of the plan.

E The evaluation of the plan.

R The reassessment.

In process recording, each contact between the nurse and the client is recorded using the format described above. Whenever possible the length of the relationship is agreed upon at the beginning of the interaction. For instance, if the client is attending an antenatal clinic, the date for completion would be determined by her expected date of delivery. In an acute surgical ward, the date of discharge may be predicted, whereas in a psychiatric setting the final date may be more fluid and agreed upon at a later date in the relationship.

Because of the different approach that would be used for assessment in this example, the recording of information would take a much less structured approach. In its simplest form, all that is required is a blank sheet of paper. However, it is sometimes helpful to have some sort of guidance to record biographical data and a sheet for use in the process system. Figure 10.3 is an example of a record which may be suitable.

Although there is no formal pattern to follow, it may be useful for the nurse to develop a framework which she can use as a mental check list during the orientation phase to ensure that there is an opportunity to discuss areas of human need which could give rise to difficulties. Needs have been written about by many people. For instance, Maslow (1954) describes a hierarchy of needs while Henderson (1966) describes 14 activities of daily living which she considers incorporate human needs. The choice may be left with the individual nurse or with the team as to which approach is taken and may vary according to the type of clinical setting and the emphasis of care. Whichever framework is chosen, it would be important that it is shared with all team members in order to facilitate communication.

WARD:	Admission Date:

Name: *Age:*
Address: *Occupation:*

Religion:

Tel. No.   *Likes to be*
                     referred to as:

Next of Kin: *Meaningful others:*
Name:
Address:

Tel. No.:

Home supports:

Medical Care:
Consultant: *Ward doctor:*
Proposed medical regime:

Date/Time	Notes	Signature
S		
O		
A		
P		

Fig. 10.3 *An assessment form.*

In the case of Mr Smith, the orientation phase may begin by discussing the circumstances which have led him to seek help. In his case, an activities of living framework may be a useful guide to the discussion. Figure 10.4 is an example of the information gathered about his nutritional needs using the process recording format.

In this example Mr Smith is able to identify his difficulties quite clearly and the orientation phase or understanding of the difficulty can be established rapidly. In other instances, this phase may take a considerable length of time with repeated interactions and recordings of the process. Even though the difficulties he found have been identified initially for Mr Smith, further assessment may reveal more information particularly as the trust develops between the two people concerned, that is the client and the nurse.

	Nursing Notes	
Date/Time	Notes	Signature
2/7/85 10 a.m. (admission interview)	S Is worried about not being able to cook own meals.	
	Says he has lost weight recently.	
	Dislikes food cooked by neighbours or provided by Meals-on-wheels.	
	Dislikes having to ask other people for help.	
	Has no appetite since he has not been able to cook own food. Cooking for him was 'part of eating'.	
	Worried about how he will cope in future.	
	O Looks thin and anxious. Can explain his own difficulties well. Dietary intake insufficient to maintain weight.	
	A Weight 9 st 1 lb (from 9 st 11 lb in May). Unable to hold heavy objects in hands, e.g. saucepans and kettle.	
	Cannot manipulate objects requiring fine movements, e.g. tin opener.	
	Currently has Meals-on-wheels on Tuesdays and Fridays. Home help cooks on other days and leaves a meal for weekends.	

Fig. 10.4 *A care plan item.*

Progressing to the identification or planning stage, Peplau suggests that, since the nurse has expert knowledge she has the major responsibility for suggesting a plan of action. Continuing to use the process format, both goals and plans may be recorded together. Figure 10.5 shows a plan for Mr Smith.

Unlike some of the other approaches that have been discussed, in this instance the information is recorded on a continual basis, a summary of each contact following the same format. However, as the care progresses, the emphasis of recording will move more towards gathering information about evaluation, and reassessment to see whether the need for nursing has been resolved and the relationship can be discontinued.

Date/Time	Nursing Notes Notes	Signature
	P Goal — Will learn to cook simple meals and hot drinks independently.	
	Refer to occupational therapist for a. advice on suitable aids b. teaching in use of aids	
	Practise use of aids in ward kitchen at least once each day.	
	Goal — Will maintain current weight.	
	Discuss diet and help to draw up a weekly menu which can be prepared independently.	
	Weigh every Friday at 9.00 a.m. in pyjamas.	
	Goal — Will gather information and understanding of services which may be helpful in the future.	
	Discuss possibility of weekly visits to social meeting at disabled centre.	
	Provide information and costing of sheltered housing.	
	Arrange for consultation of social worker.	

Fig. 10.5 *Planning care.*

A patient care study

Since process recording is obviously a continual operation, only excerpts of the care study are shown below in order to demonstrate the technique. The person concerned is a 68 year old gentleman, Mr Jack Fieldson, who has recently been widowed. He retired from his work as an architect two years ago and lost his wife six months ago. Over the last six months, he has become progressively more withdrawn and depressed and is now no longer able to care for himself. During the orientation phase of nursing, the interactions between Mr Fieldson and the nurse are aimed towards both of them learning more about the nature of Mr Fieldson's difficulties, recognising the cause of the difficulties and developing trust and understanding between them.

The professional schooling of the nurse should enable her to manage her own reactions towards this withdrawn, unresponsive gentleman and to use interactional skills in trying to help him. This should be done without over-involvement but with a professional closeness. A summary of the initial interaction is shown in Figure 10.6, followed by a further summary of the interaction which occurred five days later (Figure 10.7).

WARD: Peplau	Admission Date: 3/11/84

Name: Mr Jack Fieldson	*Age:* 68 yrs DOB: 02.07.16
Address: The Old Barn	*Occupation:* Retired architect
Mewby on the Hill	
	Religion: Baptist
	Likes to be
Tel. No.: Mewby 307	*referred to as:* Mr Fieldson

Next of Kin: Daughter	*Meaningful others:*
Name: Mrs Hilary James	Grandchildren — Kathy (6), John (4)
Address: Box Cottage	Mr and Mrs Trevor (neighbours)
Hawkesbury	
Northumberland	Tel. Mewby 362
Tel. No.: Hawkesbury 3762	

Home supports:
    Private home help 3 days weekly
    GP — family friend

Medical Care:

Consultant: Dr Everett	*Ward doctor:* John Reeves

Proposed medical regime:
    For close observation and supervision (suicide risk)
    Drug therapy

Nursing Notes (Excerpt of notes on 1st day of admission)

Date/Time		Notes	Signature
3/11/84 11 a.m.	S	Says he is worried and disturbed by being here and doesn't want to discuss the situation.	
	O	Reluctant to talk. Looking down at the floor. Wringing hands. Physically unkempt.	
	A	Is withdrawn Ashamed at being in psychiatric hospital Unable to establish any rapport at this stage.	
	P	Introduce to other patients Show ward/bed areas. Give time to familiarise himself with environment and see the doctor.	
3 p.m.	E	No change in behaviour.	
	S	Says he has seen the doctor and knows he is depressed but nothing can help. 'This place will make me even worse'.	

O   Still withdrawn avoiding eye
    contact.
    No conversation initiated with
    either staff or patients.
    Food on jacket, shirt and
    around mouth.
    Reluctant to join other patients

A   Apathetic and unhappy.
    In need of constant observation.

P   Re-interview on evening shift.
    Observe closely.

Fig. 10.6 *Biographical data and initial nursing notes.*

Date-Time		Notes	Signature
8/11/84 1 p.m.	S	Monosyllabic responses to conversation only.	
	O	Silent tears during lunch.	
		No food eaten.	
		Answers direct questions appropriately but monosyllabically. Does not express any feelings.	
		No movement around ward except when led.	
		No concern for hygiene or appearance.	
	A	Low mood worsening. Suicide risk currently reduced through apathy.	
	P	Review at multidisciplinary team meeting this afternoon.	
	I	Discussed at meeting. Patient not present.	
		Not responding to drug therapy yet. Further action needed.	
		Intensive nursing care. Continuous observation with interaction every 2 hours, or in response to non- verbal approaches, with primary nurse.	

Fig. 10.7 *Nursing notes, five days after admission.*

The first excerpt from Mr Fieldson's progress notes demonstrates the beginning phases of the development of a relationship between client and nurse. Rather than following a formal structure, both the length and initial contact are guided by Mr Fieldson's own responses to the situation and, as can be seen, in this beginning stage, the trust which is sought has not yet been established nor has the part that each of the participants will play.

During the second excerpt, the freedom of this approach is again shown. For example, although the frequency of the interactions between Mr Fieldson and his primary nurse are stated, no length of time is prescribed since this would be determined by him. However, in different circumstances, it would be quite feasible to include more details if required. The intensity of the relationship and the strain that is placed on the nurse in being in such close proximity with someone whose mood is so low is also acknowledged in that the work of observing may be shared among other members of the team, while the direct interaction would occur with the primary nurse.

At first sight it may be difficult to see how this approach can be used in settings where the major need has arisen through a physiological disorder. However, the underlying belief in developing a trusting relationship can only be seen as valuable. The approach could be particularly useful in terminal care, in fields where the emphasis of care is towards health education, and in work with the disabled. In all these areas it is particularly important that an understanding can develop between both parties and that shared learning of each other's strengths and needs can occur.

11 | Using a Nursing Model

The purpose of this last chapter of the book is to draw together all of the issues that have been raised and to offer some ideas about choosing a model and implementing it in practice. Without such action, the world of nursing can only become more confusing.

To summarise the essence of the book, an understanding and application of model-based practice will:

- Clarify the meaning of nursing.
- Identify the value system on which nursing is based.
- Give direction to practice.
- Identify the role that the nurse should fulfil.
- Allow individual nurses to be accountable for their own practice.
- Justify the nurses' contribution in a multidisciplinary clinical team.
- Point out what knowledge is needed for effective practice.
- Highlight areas of practice where research is required.
- Require that nurses have some freedom in choosing which model they should practise from.
- Guide the development of the curriculum for courses in nursing.
- Be the essential first step in trying to establish the nursing process in any nursing team.
- Lead to radical changes in the style of nursing care.

Having read the basis of these points in the preceding chapters and if these points are accepted by the reader, then the logical question to address now is 'what to do about it'. The very few nurses who work alone need to consider the nature of nursing models and to arrive at a decision about a framework on which to base their practice. They then need to incorporate this framework into their work. However, the majority of nurses work in teams in either wards, departments or community health centres. Inevitably the path they need to follow is a little different in that they will have to talk about ideas and models within the team and make a collective choice about which model to implement.

Choosing a model for practice

Before the nursing team can choose a model to practise from, it is obvious that they will need opportunities to explore various options and to discuss personal models held by individuals within the team. So the first step in choosing a model is to learn about what models for nursing practice are and why they are needed. This book aims at helping nurses in this respect, but learning about topics such as this is often easier in groups where ideas can be shared and issues clarified through pooling of understanding. In our experience, organising group meetings for staff with the purpose of studying various approaches to nursing is often far more productive than one imagines.

Such meetings offer the opportunity for team members to express their personal views and feelings and discuss those of their colleagues. A whole nursing team seldom has the opportunity of meeting together in this way, and enabling this to occur is essential because both points of arguments and agreements can be identified. Often much less agreement exists than is apparent at first sight, and finding a common solution is the beginning of moving towards model-based practice. A useful approach to take in such meetings is to ask the group to consider their own personal views on each of the three components of the model they use for their practice, namely:

- Their own views about people.
- The goals of their practice.
- The knowledge they have and the knowledge they need to achieve those goals.

Nurses who work in a specific ward, a community 'patch' or a particular department will therefore need to plan and make time for a number of nursing team meetings. The team of nurses must come to some agreement on beliefs and values; the goals of nursing; and what they all need to know, feel and be skilled in in order to achieve these goals. Then they may choose to set up some multidisciplinary team meetings. In later meetings with nurses, it is helpful to continue to discuss each other's views and to then compare the individual views on the nature of nursing models. This book will start to provide background knowledge and understanding for the group to draw on.

Through taking this approach, it is usually possible to finally agree on a set of valued beliefs, on common goals and on an outline of knowledge, skills and attitudes which the team see as fundamental to nursing practice. Sometimes this will match almost exactly a specific nursing model which has been described by others. For example, one ward which we are familiar with feels that the model developed by Orem (1980) clearly represents real nursing to them and they now use it as a basis for their practice; another has done the same with King's model (King, 1971); and another has chosen the activities of living model developed by Roper, Logan and Tierney (1980). Of course there are countless other wards which we do not know about which have selected other specific models.

Some teams find that one model does not adequately describe reality to them and they decide on an amalgamation of ideas taken from two or more models. Another ward we know of uses the activities of living as a framework for assessment, and applies stress adaptation from Roy's perspective (1976) to these activities; a district nursing team has agreed that nursing to them can only be accurately described by combining the concepts of Orem, Roper *et al.* and Roy. A team of nurses on a psychiatric ward found that none of the models meant much to them and decided that it is too early in their thinking to develop a full blown one for themselves. They have some agreement on the beliefs and values which underlie 'good' practice in the wards, on some overall goals to be achieved, and on some basic knowledge, skills and attitudes that they would like all nurses on the ward to share. All of these approaches are quite acceptable.

We are also familiar with a number of nursing teams who have not yet approached their work by considering its essence, and it is often apparent in the sort of nursing work carried out. For example, a number of teams using the 'nursing process' have developed assessment forms following the working party approach. This common approach consists of getting together a small group of staff from the centre and from the peripheral units of the Health District. They then proceed to attempt to produce some recommendations applicable to the whole district which everyone else is then supposed to agree with. In the case of the nursing process such working parties have been set up to design what are seen as the all important forms. All of the members sit around a table and suggest, for example, what headings or questions should go on the assessment form. One may suggest:

Does he/she have false teeth?

And another may develop this and urge that this be rephrased to:

Dentures: upper/lower

The end result is a form with headings and questions. This is then printed and sent to nurses throughout the district who are told to use them as a standard nursing record. When this occurs, the nursing teams are said to be 'doing the nursing process'. However, without agreement on what the *nursing* component of the process consists of, often the only change achieved in this approach is different paperwork, and there is no real change in practice.

Starting off by agreeing on a model for nursing, rather than concentrating on documentation, is far more in line with the philosophy of the nursing process. It is often less time-consuming than a district-wide working party, because a model gives clear

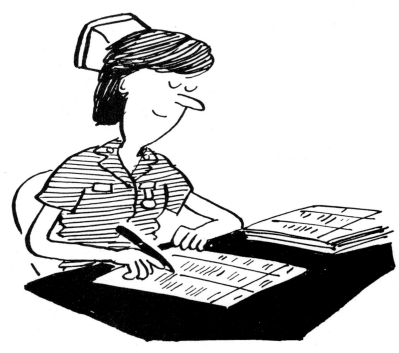

Fig. 11.1 *'Doing' the nursing process!*

structure to assessment and can be undertaken by individual teams. More importantly, however, it leads to a meaningful consideration of how care by nurses is given, and to actual and beneficial changes in practice. The working party approach leads to no more than a new nursing record, and little chance of any difference in what actually happens to patients. So choosing a model must begin from discussion and education, and is fundamental to introducing changes in nursing practice.

Students and pupil nurses do not have the opportunity to become as involved in this process as nurses who are permanently working in set areas. Therefore they usually need to be aware of the nature, basic structure of and the differences between various models. It is important, however, for student or pupil nurses, to sort out their own views and choose something which falls in with them. The rotation around clinical units gives them a unique opportunity to see how various teams nurse, and how they apply their own model to patient care.

Choosing a nursing model is *not* like choosing a new carpet or a dish from the menu of an exclusive restaurant. Such things are 'one off' and once the choice is made, that is it. Choosing a model demands a close scrutiny of ourselves, our patients, other nurses and other health workers. It is not a choice from which there is no going back. As new ideas arrive, new concepts are identified, and patients' needs change, so then does the possible choice of model change.

When you buy a new coat 'you pays your money and takes your chance' may well apply, but choosing a model is merely the beginning in a whole cobweb-like chain of ever-growing choices.

Implementing a nursing model in practice

If a nursing team finds that it can agree that a certain model represents nursing and that it should form the basis for practice, it is then possible to implement its use within the team.

To introduce this new perspective into the work situation is, in effect, to implement change. Much is written about how to introduce change and a number of theories exist. For a deeper analysis of the change process and strategy for change we direct you to the wealth of literature available elsewhere. We simply want to outline the basis for change and relate this to introducing model-based practice by suggesting the approach we have used.

Change refers to the process which brings about alteration in behaviour or substitutes one way of behaviour for another. Some changes occur because of things around us, but most changes cannot effectively occur without being planned. Planned change is inevitably easier to manage than change which is imposed, haphazard or misunderstood. Nursing in itself can be seen to be an agent of change. It hopes to bring about changes in patients' or clients' behaviour, such as changing dependence into independence, fear into security and so forth. We all know the argument that planned nursing care is more effective than unplanned care, hence the current emphasis in nursing on the use of problem solving. The four steps used in problem solving or the nursing process are useful in providing a framework to plan change. So, in introducing the model of your choice into practice, it is useful to consider it under the following headings:

Assessment

First of all one needs to assess the situation: what is the current situation? Who will be involved in using the model? Who will it affect? What changes will it require in such things as work organisation, duty rotas and so on? What resources will be needed, such as new assessment, care planning and evaluation documents? Are these resources available? If so, how can they be obtained, and if not what can be done about it? What needs to be done to overcome problems which will inhibit the introduction of the changes? For example, if lack of understanding by some of the nurses or doctors, physiotherapists, and domestics is apparent, it may be that the opportunity for learning is necessary before the desired change in practice can be made acceptable to them.

Planning

Having identified the problem, a plan of action can be prepared. For example, the appropriate assessment forms can be ordered; group discussions and teaching can be arranged to give a greater understanding of the model, and perhaps the use of the assessment framework. If lack of skills and knowledge or disparity in attitudes in the team have been identified as problems, plans for educational experiences may be developed to overcome them. Meetings with the multidisciplinary clinical team may also be planned. The plan may include target dates for introduction of specific changes and for evaluating them. Incorporated into the plan must also be some means by which the effects of the change will be evaluated. In this way success can actually be measured leading to encouragement and satisfaction for the nurses concerned.

Implementation

In this step the plan is actually put into action, and the change is regularly monitored, by previously agreed methods, to judge its effectiveness. In the area where one of us works this approach was taken. The nursing team was given the opportunity to express their own views, learn about a variety of nursing models and select the one which they felt closest to. They then planned for educational sessions themselves. These were designed to enable them to become skilled in communicating with patients and to discover and revise their own attitudes to patient care. In addition to these sessions, they planned to meet with the doctors, social workers, physiotherapists and occupational therapists to describe the model and to negotiate the right within the multidisciplinary clinical team that nursing has to work in this way and to clarify how this would affect the work and relationships between disciplines.

Evaluation

This plan was implemented and on evaluation, patients, nurses and the multidisciplinary clinical team had a greater understanding of nursing itself. Patients became more independent and the average length of stay in the wards was reduced. The multidisciplinary clinical team valued the contribution of nursing more highly, with many admissions to the ward being regarded by the team as being best served if the patient's nurse became leader of the multi-disciplinary team. The nurses indicated that they were more satisfied with their role than before.

Change never, of course, runs smoothly and perhaps this description sounds simple and easy. The actual process we describe, however, seems to be the only way of effectively introducing any change, and that includes introducing the use of a model for practice.

Choosing a model and implementing it in practice is, we believe, crucial to the provision of nursing care at a standard we would like to receive for ourselves, our family or our friends, if the need for nursing were ever to arise.

Implications for nurse education

Inevitably a shift from one model of practice to another will be of major concern to those nurses working in nurse education. Examination of the curricula of the 1950s and 1960s clearly demonstrates that the implicit model for practice was the biomedical model where the orientation was towards disease and cure. Many of us can vividly remember this emphasis from our own training. Yet a shift is now occurring away from a disease-centred orientation or medical model curriculum towards a client-centred orientation or nursing model curriculum. In a recent study of 270 American schools, De Back (1981) was unable to find any which still based their curricula on the medical model, which she described as 'organised around disease processes'. The most commonly identified or popular framework was a systems model approach that is 'organised around stability and adaptation of the client'. While to the best of our knowledge no such evidence exists in this country at the moment, such a shift is nevertheless also occurring, as reflected by, as mentioned earlier, the change in emphasis in the 1982 RNMH syllabus.

Torres and Yura (1974) discuss how the model of choice for a particular practice discipline is reflected in the curriculum. They portray a model or conceptual framework as containing theories which reflect the philosophy, goals and desired behaviour for practice. (See Figure 11.2.) They continue to describe how such a framework can be used in curriculum design, identifying six stages to this end.

- Statement of the philosophy of the programme.
- The broad objectives of the programme.
- The statement of the terminal behaviour flowing from the programme.
- The outline of the conceptual framework.

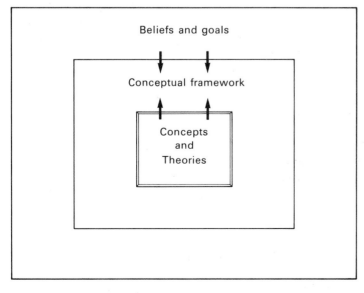

Fig. 11.2 *Curriculum design components.*

These initial stages will provide a rationale for the selection of learning experience and a system for classifying knowledge and ordering facts. Once this has been achieved the educator will:

- Develop the level behavioural statements required for each stage of the course.
- Designate the learning experience needed to meet these objectives.

The shift from a disease-centred to a client-centred model has obvious implications for nurse educators not only in the content of what they teach, but also in the methods that they employ in their teaching. If there is an emphasis on the patient as an individual, with a right to participate in his or her own decision making, then there is an implication that the same belief should be reflected in the nurse educator's relationship with the student or pupil.

One of the points that has been emphasised throughout this book is that there is no right or wrong model and that individual nurses have the right to choose which one they will base their practice on. Even if they work in a team of nurses, they can contribute their ideas to the group decision. It has also been stressed that it is essential for a curriculum to be based on an explicit model: indeed it is impossible to develop a curriculum without some kind of conceptual framework.

These two points can create a very difficult dilemma for nurse educators to which there is no simple answer. During their clinical secondments, students and pupils will be faced with working in a number of different settings, all of which will be using a different model base. If the belief that clinical nurses have the right to choose their own model for practice is accepted then, in the current apprenticeship-type system of nurse training and education, learners will inevitably be exposed to numerous different approaches to care. Yet, it has also been suggested that the curriculum should be devised around a specific model.

Several solutions have been offered as a way of overcoming this difficulty, none of which has proved right or wrong. We can only put forward some of the ideas and leave you to make your own judgement about their merits and deficits.

First, some schools have taken a very eclectic approach, amalgamating ideas from various different models which they believe to be important. In other words they have attempted to develop a single unified model of their own.

A second approach has been to choose a single model on which to base the curriculum. The ideas of other models may be raised but the direction of the curriculum would be based on one. Undoubtedly from a curriculum design stance, this is the most satisfactory answer. However, it does raise difficulties in transferring learning to working in settings where a different framework from that used in the curriculum is practised.

A third approach is to divide the curriculum into different components and teach each component using a specific model. For instance, one year may be devoted to learning about the nursing needs of patients who are affected by 'episodic illness', during which a systems approach such as that described by Roy could be used. Another year may deal with the nursing needs of patients requiring continuing care, and a curriculum based on a developmental approach such as that described by Peplau could be used. The framework for the curriculum could be chosen to reflect the one most commonly used in the relevant clinical area.

Whichever approach is chosen, the important thing is that learners are introduced to the idea of models for practice and how they affect their work.

Implications for nurse managers

Many of the problems which face nurse educators will also affect nurse managers. The management structure which has traditionally been employed in nursing is that of the bureaucracy, based on a hierarchical system with clearly stated rules and regulations or policies which say what nurses can or cannot do according to their level or status.

Model-based practice implies that it is the individual practitioners or the teams they work in which control the way in which they work. From a management perspective this raises two dilemmas. While managers have the responsibility for ensuring that the organisation fulfils the purpose for which it is designed, that is to supply a nursing service, they have little control of *how* that service is supplied. Provided that the standards which have been established are fulfilled, *the way* in which these standards are reached may vary from setting to setting according to which model the practice is based on. Inevitably this will alter the function of the manager from one of controller to one of facilitator — a much more exacting role to fulfil. Much more flexibility may be needed in setting policies in order to allow for individual variations in different settings. For instance, if the goals of a ward are geared towards independence, it would be inappropriate to make a rule about the use of cot sides for elderly patients. Similarly in a community setting, no rule could be set about the time by which all morning insulins must be given if they are to be planned on an individual basis.

So, if a manager's role in controlling the way in which nurses practise is reduced, what is their function? We would see them developing and expanding their role as facilitator, with a much greater emphasis on providing the facilities which allow clinical nurses to practise. This may involve such things as providing learning opportunities, assessing standards and dependency levels, and ensuring that services and equipment are available, as well as providing the essential moral support for clinical colleagues.

This is not an easy transition, especially as many nurse managers will not have had the opportunity to practise nursing using a nursing model themselves. Yet it can also offer a new and exciting dimension to their work and the satisfaction of seeing improved patient care.

Implications for nursing research

There has been a rapid increase in the amount of nursing research being carried out over the last ten years, both by nurses in formal research posts and by clinical nurses themselves. One of the most difficult things to do in research is to define the exact nature of the problem in question, and it is in this area that models of nursing can be so useful.

As we are sure you know by now, models are based on philosophies or beliefs and goals which reflect theories and concepts. Research is about testing ideas in order to acquire new knowledge. Putting these two thoughts together, the direction of research may be either:

• To refine theories *of* nursing — what are the related concepts? How do they relate to each other and to nursing itself? Is there an alternative model of nursing?
• To refine theories *for* nursing. If I do this or that, will it be useful in helping patients to achieve their goals? In using a model, deficits in the knowledge required for practice can be identified.

Working from a model base can help in clarifying either of these two aspects of research, giving it purpose and direction. We know of several clinically-based nurses who have developed excellent small scale research based on a conceptual framework which is clearly nursing in nature. For instance, one clinical nurse examined whether teaching relaxation to people reduces the number of tension-induced symptoms they suffer (Newing, 1985). Another looked at what problems patients face in fulfilling activities of living following the stress of surgery, regardless of what the surgery is for. It is clear that an explicit model of nursing can contribute significantly to the work of those nurses undertaking research.

Conclusion

In this book we have attempted to introduce you to the ideas inherent in model-based practice. While the first four chapters were largely theoretical in nature, outlining the common characteristics of nursing models, we feel that they are an essential background to the practical use of models. Other chapters have tried to show you how the theory can be applied through presenting practical illustrations based on specific nursing models. It is at this stage that we can hand the work over to you. Nobody can tell you which model to choose or how to implement it. If we presumed to try to tell you, we would be going against our own beliefs in an individual's right to make choices for him or herself. The model we agree on tells us that this is the way we should behave!

We cannot pretend that it is easy to either identify the model relevant to your work or to put it into practice. All we can say is that in our opinion the path is worth following.

Science is built up with facts as a house is with stones, but a collection of facts is no more a science than a heap of stones is a house.

Jules Henri Poincare, *La Science et l'Hypothese*

References and Bibliography

Apple D. (1960). How laymen define illness. *Journal of Health and Human Behaviour*; **1(3):** 219–25.

Bauman B. (1961). Diversities in conceptions of health and physical fitness. *Journal of Health and Human Behaviour*; **2(1):** 39–46.

Bennett J. G. (1980). Foreword to symposium on the self-care concept of nursing. *Nursing Clinics of North America*; **15:1.** Philadelphia: W. B. Saunders.

Bevis E. O. (1978). *Curriculum Building in Nursing*. St. Louis: C. V. Mosby.

Byrne M., Thompson L. (1978). *Key concepts for the study and practice of nursing*, 2nd edn. St. Louis: C. V. Mosby.

Capra F. (1982). *The Turning Point: Science, Society and the Rising Culture*. London: Fontana Paper Backs.

Chin R. (1980). The utility of systems models and developmental models for practitioners. In *Conceptual Models for Nursing Practice*, 2nd edn. (Riehl J. P., Roy C., eds.). New York: Appleton Century Crofts.

Craddock R. B., Stanhope N. K. (1980). The Neuman Health Care Systems Model: Recommended Adaptations. In *Conceptual Models for Nursing Practice*, 2nd edn. (Riehl J. P., Roy C., eds.). New York: Appleton Century Crofts.

Davis F. (1975). Professional socialisation as subjective experience: the process of doctrinal conversion among student nurses. In *A sociology of medical practice* (Cox C., Mead A., eds.). London: Collier MacMillan.

De Back V. (1981). The relationship between senior nursing students' ability for formulating nursing diagnoses and curriculum model. *A.N.S.*; **3(3):** 51–66

De Cecco J. D., Crawford W. R. (1974). *The Psychology of learning and instruction*, 2nd edn. Old Tappan, New Jersey: Prentice Hall.

Field D. (1972). Disability as social deviance. In *Medical men and their work* (Friedson E., Corber J., eds.). New York: Aldine Atherton.

Friedson E. (1975). *Profession of Medicine*. New York: Dodd, Mead and Co.

General Nursing Council for England and Wales (1982). *Training Syllabus, Register of Nurses, Mental Subnormality Nursing*. London: GNC.

Glaser R. (1962). Psychology and Instructional Technology. In *Training Resources and Education* (Glaser R., ed.). Pittsburgh: University of Pittsburgh Press.

Henderson V. (1966). *The Nature of Nursing*. London: Collier Mac-Millan.

Illich I. (1975). *Medical Nemesis*. Harmondsworth: Pelican.

Joseph L. S. (1980). Self care and the nursing process. *Nursing Clinics of North America*; **15:1**. Philadelphia: W. B. Saunders.

King I. M. (1971). *Toward a theory for nursing*. New York: John Wiley.

Kübler-Ross E. (1969). *On death and dying*. London: Tavistock.

Levin L., Katz A., Holst E. (1979). *Self-care: lay initiatives in health*. New York: Prodist.

Lewis F. M., Batey M. V. (1982). Clarifying autonomy and accountability in nursing service – part II. *Journal of Nursing Administration*; **12(10):** 10–15.

Maslow A. H. (1954). *Motivation and Personality*. New York: Harper & Row.

McFarlane J. (1978). *The multi-disciplinary clinical team*. London: King's Fund.

Mullin V. J. (1981). Implementing the self-care concept in the acute care setting. *Nursing Clinics of North America*; **15.1**. Philadelphia: W. B. Saunders.

Neuman B. (1980). The Betty Neuman Health Care Systems Model: A total approach to patient problems. In *Conceptual Models for Nursing Practice*, 2nd edn. (Riehl J., Roy C., eds.). New York: Appleton Century Croft.

Neuman B., Wyatt M. (1981). Prospects for change: some evaluative reflections from one articulated baccalaureate program. *Journal of Nursing Education*; January **20(1):** 40–6.

Neuman B., Young R. J. (1972). A model for teaching total person approach to patient problems. *Nursing Research*; **21(3):** 264.

Neuman B. (1982). *The Neuman Systems Model*. New York: Appleton Century Croft.

Newing M. (1985). *Group processes: a subjective exploration*. Oxford: Burford Nursing Development Unit.

Norris C. M. (1979). Self care. *American Journal of Nursing*; **79(3):** 486–9.

Nursing Development Conference Group (1973). *Concept Formulization in Nursing*, Boston: Little, Brown and Co.

Orem D. (1980). *Nursing — concepts of practice*, 2nd edn. New York: McGraw Hill.

Parsons T. (1951). *The Social System*. London: Routledge & Kegan Paul.

Pearson A. (1983). *The Clinical Nursing Unit*. London: William Heinemann Medical Books.

Pearson A., Vaughan B. (1984). Module I: Nursing practice and the nursing process. In *A Systematic Approach to Nursing Care — an introduction*. Milton Keynes: Open University.

Peplau H. E. (1980). The psychiatric nurse — accountable? to whom? for what? *Perspectives in Psychiatric Care*; **18(3):** 128–34.

Peplau H. E. (1969). Professional closeness. *Nursing Forum*; **8(4):** 342–60.

Peplau H. E. (1952). *Interpersonal relations in nursing*. New York: G. P. Putman.

Piaget J. (1932). *The Moral Judgement of the Child*. London: Routledge & Kegan Paul.

Pietroni P. (1984). Holistic Medicine. New Map, Old Territory. *The British Journal of Holistic Medicine*; **1:** 3–13.

Rambo B. J. (1984). *Adaptation nursing: assessment and intervention*. Philadelphia: W. B. Saunders.

Rogers M. (1970). *An introduction to the theoretical basis of nursing*. Philadelphia: F. A. Davis.

Roper N. (1976). *Clinical Experience in Nurse Education*. Edinburgh: Churchill Livingstone.

Roper N., Logan W., Tierney A. (1981). *Learning to Use the Process of Nursing*. Edinburgh: Churchill Livingstone.

Roper N., Logan W., Tierney A. (1980). *The Elements of Nursing*. Edinburgh: Churchill Livingstone.

Rose A. M. (1980). A systematic summary of symbolic interaction theory. In *Conceptual Models for Nursing Practice*, 2nd edn. (Riehl J. P., Roy C., eds.). New York: Appleton Century Croft.

Roy C. (1976). *Inroduction to Nursing: An Adaptation Model*. Old Tappan, New Jersey: Prentice Hall.

Royal Commission on the National Health Service (1978). *Patient Attitudes to the Hospital Service*. Norwich: HMSO.

Russell B. (1961). *History of Western Philosophy*. London: Allen & Unwin.

Selye H. (1978). *The stress of life*. New York: McGraw Hill.

Sills G. M. (1978). Hildegard E. Peplau: Leader, practitioner, academic, scholar and theorist. *Perspectives in Psychiatric Care*; **16(3):** 22–28.

Smuts J. C. (1926). *Holism and Evolution*. New York: MacMillan.

Stevenson L. (1974). *Seven Theories of Human Nature*. Oxford: Oxford University Press.

Torres G., Yura H. (1974). Today's conceptual framework: its relationship to the curriculum development process. *National League for Nursing Publ*; **15–1529:** 1–12.

World Health Organisation (1948). *Constitution*. Geneva: WHO.

Index